Advance Praise for
Culture AND THE Condom

"Heads up, colleagues: this book is a perfect and timely hands-on manual that will certainly grab your attention."

John Weaver, Georgia Southern University

"Karen Anijar and Thuy DaoJensen have given us a hugely important...and at times entertaining...book. It's about condoms, yes, but also about how we think about sex, sexuality, and the legislation of both."

David Gabbard, East Carolina University

"This is an important book that is about much more than condoms. It speaks to important issues in the popular culture that have been generally ignored or under-discussed."

Thomas Barone, Arizona State University

Culture
AND THE
Condom

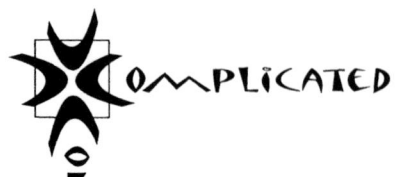

A Book Series of
Curriculum Studies

William F. Pinar
General Editor

VOLUME 10

PETER LANG
New York • Washington, D.C./Baltimore • Bern
Frankfurt am Main • Berlin • Brussels • Vienna • Oxford

Culture
AND THE
Condom

Karen Anijar & Thuy DaoJensen, EDITORS

PETER LANG
New York • Washington, D.C./Baltimore • Bern
Frankfurt am Main • Berlin • Brussels • Vienna • Oxford

Library of Congress Cataloging-in-Publication Data

Culture and the condom / edited by Karen Anijar, Thuy DaoJensen.
    p. cm. — (Complicated conversation; v. 10)
    Includes bibliographical references and index.
1. Sexual ethics—United States. 2. Sex instruction—United States.
3. Condoms—United States. 4. Contraception—United States.
5. Sexually transmitted diseases—Prevention—United States.
6. Sex in popular culture—United States.
7. Sexual abstinence—Religious aspects—United States.
I. Anijar, Karen. II. DaoJensen, Thuy. III. Series.
HQ32.C85   613.9'435—dc22   2005002241
ISBN 0-8204-7407-X
ISSN 1534-2816

Bibliographic information published by **Die Deutsche Bibliothek**.
Die Deutsche Bibliothek lists this publication in the "Deutsche
Nationalbibliografie"; detailed bibliographic data is available
on the Internet at http://dnb.ddb.de/.

Cover art by Adriana Bertini
Cover design by Sophie Boorsch Appel

© 2005 Peter Lang Publishing, Inc., New York
275 Seventh Avenue, 28th Floor, New York, NY 10001
www.peterlangusa.com

All rights reserved.
Reprint or reproduction, even partially, in all forms such as microfilm,
xerography, microfiche, microcard, and offset strictly prohibited.

CONTENTS

Acknowledgments vii

Foreword by Peter McLaren ix

Chapter One: Abstinence Makes the Heart Grow Fonder:
Christians, Condoms, Curriculum, and Apocalyptic Sexuality 1
   by Karen Anijar

Chapter Two: When Condoms Go Bad:
From Safe Sex to Five Microns to *Killer Condom* 21
   by Thuy DaoJensen

Chapter Three: Queer Eye on the Straight Guy's Condoms 29
   by Jessamyn Neuhaus

Chapter Four: Making Condoms Transgressive:
South Park and "Proper Condom Use" 37
   by Mary M. Dalton

Chapter Five: Don't Avoid or Make Void the Topic 49
   by Chris Bell

Chapter Six: Exchanging Fluid Discourses of Social Dis-ease:
Visual Cultural Studies as Prophylactic Praxis as Rough Trade 59
   by James H. Sanders

Chapter Seven: Condoms, Penis Size, and Statistics:
One Size Definitely Does Not Fit All! 77
   by Michael J. Nanna

Chapter Eight: The Condom in History: Shame and Fear 93
   by Mark Lipton

Chapter Nine: Stiff Competition: A Thrust for Condom Education 105
   by Devon C. Adams

Chapter Ten: Engineering the Condom 109
    by Charla Triplett

Chapter Eleven: Sanctioned Discourse: Women, Condoms,
and HIV/AIDS in Early 1990s Government Brochures 117
    by Dacia Charlesworth

Chapter Twelve: Female Identity and the Construction of
Condom Use Among Young African-American Women 131
    by Janis Faye Hutchinson

Chapter Thirteen: Latex Condom Fashions 163
    by Thuy DaoJensen

Chapter Fourteen: The Condom King 169
    by Vern L. Bullough

Chapter Fifteen: Family Planning and Male Friendships:
Sathi Condom and Same-Sex Sexual Desire Among Men
in Pakistan 177
    by Ahmed Afzal

Chapter Sixteen: The Colors of the Condom:
Benetton's Seductive Images 207
    by Jill Scott

Chapter Seventeen: Condom Flowers 229
    by Angelika Foerst

Contributors 231

Index 235

• ACKNOWLEDGMENTS •

We, the editors, are deeply indebted to many people who helped us traverse through the process of putting together this book. The production staff at Peter Lang: Justin Pelegano, Sophie Appel, and Valerie Shea, were diligent and worked tirelessly in helping us get our book ready for publication.

We wanted to thank all the authors who contributed to this book, as they provide a wide range of perspectives on the subject. Special thanks to Jessamyn Neuhaus in playing a major role in getting this project up and running, she deserves accolades for her dedication to this project.

Our project would not be alive today if not for the staff members at Arizona State University, Nancy Chavez and Valerie Craig. They have literally "dropped everything" to ensure that our project was completed. When there were obstacles to overcome, we knew we could count on them to help us every step of the way.

Finally, we would like to thank and dedicate this book to the men in our lives, Scott and Joshua (Karen's husband and son) and Troy and Colby (Thuy's husband and son).

• FOREWORD •

Peter McLaren

Shortly after waking up one morning, and while I was still in a twilight frame of mind (what anthropologists would call a *liminal* state) between sleep and consciousness, a scene played out before me that involved our beloved Attorney General, John Ashcroft. A few days before I had gone to see Michael Moore's landmark film, *Fahrenheit 9/11* and, as is often the case, I woke up thinking about the state of the world and our responsibilities for making it a better place. My usual reflections on Marxism, socialism, and grassroots activism were nudged out of frame by an arresting technicolor image of John Ashcroft, wearing his trademark all-American smile and marching in a Fourth of July parade. Dressed as Uncle Sam, he was walking on stilts and singing his signature song, the blockbuster Pentecostal paen, *Let the Eagle Soar*. Then the scene began suddenly to shift. Following the ritual he has performed each time he has been sworn into office, he asks to be anointed with cooking oil (in the manner of King David). Pushing his top hat jauntily to one side so that I might apply unimpeded some Crisco oil to his forehead, I notice that his skin is the texture of latex, and that he is actually wearing over his head a John Ashcroft condom. I glance below at his flabalance and notice that below the equator he is brandishing a large Statue of Liberty codpiece. Our (presumably) tumescent Attorney General seems oblivious to the shocked looks on the faces of the suburban families who have lined the streets to enjoy the parade, listen to the Attorney General's rich baritone voice, and anticipate the fireworks finale.

I am relieved when the image suddenly vanishes. Was the scene a lurid enactment of the animating ideal of evangelical Christianity's "family values" revealing the hypocrisy and fanaticism that has come to define the Bush Jr. administration? Or, as Ebenezer Scrooge might put it, was it just an undigested piece of cheese that I ate the night before? In either case, it brings up one of the pervasive themes of this volume: that the right to live is supernumerary relative to the shaping of American values by leaders in the thrall of evangelical Christian fanaticism and the value form of labor wrought by capitalism.

It has been well-documented that George Bush is a devout evangelical Christian who claimed that God directed him to invade Iraq. Bush unhesitatingly made his decision to invade and occupy Iraq "because he believes, he truly believes, that God squats in his brainpan and tells him what to do" (Floyd, 2003, p. 4). The Israeli newspaper *Haaretz* was given transcripts of a negotiating session between former Palestinian Prime Minister Mahmoud Abbas and faction leaders from Hamas and other militant groups. In these transcripts, Abbas described his recent summit with Ariel Sharon and Bush hijo. During the summit, Bush told Abbas:

> "God told me to strike at al Qaida and I struck them, and then He instructed me to strike at Saddam, which I did, and now I am determined to solve the problem in the Middle East. If you help me I will act, and if not, the elections will come and I will have to focus on them" (Regular, 2003, p. 1).

What is most frightening is the chillingly preordained character of the Bush plutocracy, given supernatural ballast by Bush's claim to be a special envoy of God. That he has asserted with clairvoyant confidence that God has appointed him president, and has called on him to lay waste to the evil-doers of the world (at least those evil-doers who sit on both untapped and fully operational oil reserves) has, for many God-fearing Christian Americans, given Bush the moral authority to turn the carnage inflicted by the world's most fearsome military machine into sacred wrath. Here the national catechism is underwritten by a fiendish commitment to capital's worldwide exponential escalation of its capacity to produce and stabilized by the incandescent belief that it is more profitable for capital intergenerationally to produce and reproduce poverty than to end poverty around the globe. God apparently regulates the world through the deregulation of the economy, where human beings are supposed to benefit from the trickle-down of capitalist self-interest.

Our priests of the capitalist era, headquartered in Washington, glibly export to the disenfranchised and oppressed a humvee pedagogy of authoritarian populism and militarism via the corporate media celebration of U.S. military firepower and congressional support for the U.S. Patriot Act.

Thanks to Bush Jr. and the corporate elite worldwide, the detritus of developed and developing security states is growing more and more visible throughout the world, as the poor continue to be exterminated by war, genocide, starvation, military and police repression, slavery, and suicide. Those whose labor-power is now deemed worthless have the choice of selling their organs, working the plantations or mines, or going into prostitution. While the United States exports its pollution to Latin America, where *maquiladoras* factories dot the border zones between the United States and Mexico, in Africa, thriving businesses sell "dead white men's clothing" in places such as the Congo, Nigeria, Lagos, Liberia, Uganda, Kenya, Tanzania, Malawi, and Togo. Here, where people survive on less than a dollar a day, on a continent that is losing its capacity to produce its own clothing, they are scrambling for Western hand-me-downs. Second-hand clothes are not the only consumer items that have turned Africa into the world's recycling bin, but also include expired medicines, antiquated computers, polluting refrigerators, air conditioners, old mattresses, and used vehicles imported from Japan (Maharaj, 2004).

The increasingly privatized public sphere gives form and substance to the unconscious avidity of the ruling elite and continues to be empowered by globalization, as corporations, financial institutions, and wealthy individuals seize more and more control. The creation of conditions favorable to private investment becomes the cardinal function of the government. Deregulation, privatization of public service, and cutbacks in public spending for social welfare are the natural outcomes of this process. The signal goal here is competitive return on investment capital. In effect, financial markets controlled by foreign investors regulate government policy and not the other way around since investment capital is for the most part outside all political control.

Of course, the era of imperialist rivalry is still with us, even though capitalism has mutated since the days of Lenin. The logic of U.S. imperialism is perhaps best captured by the way in which lobbyists, public relations counselors and confidential advisors to senior federal officials in the Bush W. administration—those very same advisors who railed against the brutality of Saddam Hussein, vociferously warned against Iraq's weapons of mass destruction, and argued that it was a supernal duty to bring freedom and democracy to Iraq—are pocketing large sums of cash for helping business clients pursue federal contracts and other financial opportunities in Iraq. But many Americans don't see this as a conflict of interest; rather, they see it as looking out for their own interests (Roche & Silverstein, 2004). After all, self-interest is what the logic of capital is all about, is it not?

Is it any wonder that little of the public sphere is still irrigable, and even less space remains to rebuild the solidarities that are such an irrefragable necessity at this particular historical juncture?

George W. Bush is clearly out to defeat the Beast of the Apocalypse. But unbeknownst to Bush, the Beast that so terrifies him and other evangelicals of his ilk does not slither through smoking corridors of fire and brimstone dragging behind it naked virgins in leather hip boots and wrapped in chains; rather, it gleefully straddles the behemoth of neoliberal capitalism, sporting a

Ronald Reagan mask and leather chaps, and digging its spurs into the flesh of the poor as it garrisons capitalism for the benefit of the transnational ruling elite, leaving in its wake worldwide empowerment of the rich and devastation for the ranks of the poor as oligopolistic corporations swallow the globe and industry becomes dominated by new technologies. It is the very behemoth that was created and is currently supported by those politicians who rule the world from positions of personal delusion, private fear, arrogance, and stupidity.

In such a world, where God is likened to a corporation, a sacerdotal entity that is legally required to put is own interests above those of everyone else, men and women are increasingly enlisted in an "us-against-them" battle royal against liberal values. It is here that Karen Anijar and Thuy DaoJensen's book, *Culture and the Condom*, takes on a singular importance. Consider the insight generated in Anijar's contribution—that the abstinence-only curriculum and the "just say no" culture of Christian conservatism helps to produce among some young adults the notion that authentic sex is heterosexual and reproductive and occurs only within the confines of marriage and therefore, anal and oral sex outside of marriage (especially if it occurs without orgasm) is not really sex and can be engaged in without protection. Approximately 38 million people are currently infected with HIV, 25 million of them live in sub-Saharan Africa and 7.2 million in Asia. Since the International AIDS Conference was held in Barcelona in 2002, 6 million people have died of AIDS and 10 million people have become newly infected, even though antiretroviral drugs have become available to more and more people infected with HIV. Most of these drugs are made by European and U.S. pharmaceutical corporations, costing as much as $5,000 per person per year, whereas generic copies of these drugs can cost as little as $150 per person per year.

While Thailand, India, and Brazil are making cheap generic drugs, not enough of the drugs are being produced to make a huge impact on effectively combating AIDS worldwide. In addition, the $15 billion over five years for AIDS treatment programs which George W. Bush has pledged to be made available through a series of bilateral agreements—known as the President's Emergency Plan for AIDS Relief—has come under fierce criticism as the United States is accused of blackmailing poor countries by asking them to relinquish rights to make the generic drugs in return for free-trade agreements (an accusation they deny). While the World Trade Organization gives developing countries the flexibility to ignore foreign patents and produce their own generic brands in times of health crises, nothing prevents a country such as the United States from imposing patent restrictions when negotiating a bilateral trade agreement. Clearly, such bilateral agreements need to be scrutinized carefully by the world community.

Currently, the money that the United States gives to AIDS research, treatment, and prevention goes to countries that support its abstinence-only policy; presently, the money can only be used to purchase brand-name drugs, because Washington has insisted that only drugs approved by the United States Food and Drug Administration can be endorsed.

Recently at the 15th International AIDS Conference in Bangkok, a controversy erupted over whether abstaining from sex or using condoms was more effective to prevent the disease. Many scientists and policy makers argue that providing condoms and clean syringes to intravenous drug users is by far the most trusted weapon in controlling the pandemic of AIDS (a philosophy they call CNN—Condoms, Needles, and Negotiating Skills), while the administration of George W. Bush argues that giving pride of place to condoms increases sexual activity among unmarried youth. The Bush administration promotes a policy known as ABC that prioritizes Abstinence, Being Faithful, and Condoms, in that order.

Ugandan President Yoweri Museveni argued at the conference that abstinence was the best way to prevent the disease, a position that mirrors the Bush Jr. administration's position. However, U.S. Congresswoman, Barbara Lee, brought up the important point that a program based on abstinence until marriage is irresponsible and inhuman because for many young women, abstaining from sex is not a choice.

While *Culture and the Condom* will not resolve these and other issues involving condom use and AIDS prevention, it offers an important context from which such debates can be engaged and deepened. That we cannot couch truth in any single predicate, least of which those that run off the tongue of evangelical politicians like Bush, and that we must examine questions of the intersection of science and religion relationally, is one of the prevailing messages of this book. While the topic of the book is the condom, the emergent themes that percolate from the pages are international in scope and tap recent debates in the fields of bioethics, religion, jurisprudence, education, and economics. The topics are wide-ranging as well, and include media representations of the condom in *Queer Eye for the Straight Guy, South Park,* and the cult film, *Killer Condom,* discussions of the abstinence-only curriculum, an analysis of Benetton's controversial condom advertisements, revelations from international condom projects and protest art, to discussions of HIV among ethnic minority populations. In this volume, we are introduced to the process of cultural production as it comes to define the meaning of the condom in various international settings. We are challenged to rethink some of our assumptions about race, gender, class, and sexuality in relation to the current campaign of AIDS prevention. This outstanding collection is cultural politics at its best. It will have a wide appeal for all those interested in the history of sexuality, gender studies, media, studies, education, sociology, and international studies.

While clearly the politics that underwrite this book will stick as uncomfortably in Bush hijo's craw as a salted pretzel, I would urge conservatives and liberals alike to engage this book. Not everyone will agree with this book, but it is imperative that they engage it.

Bibliography

Floyd, C. (2003, June 30). The Revelation of St. George. Available from: *www.counterpunch.org/floyd06302003.html*

Maharaj, D. (2004). For Sale—Cheap: 'Dead White Men's Clothing.' *Los Angeles Times,* 14 July. Available from: *www.latimes.com/news/specials/world/la-fg-clothes14jul14,1,5275395.story?coll=la-home-headlines.*

Regular, A. (2003). 'Road map is a life saver for us,' PM Abbas tells Hamas, Haaron, 11 August. Available from: *www.haaretz.com/hasen/pages/ShArt.jhtml?itemNo=310788&contrassID=2&subContrassID=1&sbSub ContrassID=0&listSrc=Y.*

Roche, W. F. and Silverstein, K. (2004). Advocates of War Now Profit from Iraq's Reconstruction. *Los Angeles Times,* 14 July. Available from:*www.latimes.com/news/nationworld/nation/la-na-advocates14jul14,0, 5891692.story.*

• CHAPTER ONE •

Abstinence Makes the Heart Grow Fonder:
Christians, Condoms, Curriculum,
and Apocalyptic Sexuality

Karen Anijar

Language is often deployed as a strategy in ideological warfare. Subjects are transformed into objects, while objects become laden with signifiers. In the battles surrounding sex education, the condom is transformed from a means of protection into the cause of a problem. In this chapter I interrogate abstinence-based sex education curricula using narratives collected from students, teachers, and parents. I situate the narratives within the content of news stories, web sites, and curricular artifacts.

My interest in the topic began when I took a group of my middle school boys (my son included) to Grauman's Chinese Theater in Los Angeles to see the movie *Outbreak*. The boys, terrified of an incurable viral outbreak (much like the one they saw in the movie), began a conversation surrounding the movie's plotline, understood within the context of their own lives and the public political pedagogy surrounding them. The discussion was punctuated with a variety of signifiers seen in the film: "AIDS," "Africa," "Mexico," "condoms," and "abstinence." These metaphors provided the foundation for their nascent adolescent sexual theorizing. Joey, one of the young men, finally said: "The truth is, if you are going to have sex, you are going to die." "Joey," I asked, "where did you learn that?" "In sex ed class," he responded. I countered: "If you use a condom, you will be protected." Daniel (another young man) replied, "No, because condoms can break." Ultimately, their conversation took on a more playful tone, as they sang, "How many condoms does it take until you are safe?" to the tune of "99 Bottles of Beer on the Wall." They also played a creative (albeit sophomoric) game of one-upmanship focusing on alternate uses for condoms, including placing them on the exhaust pipes of teachers' cars, creating art projects (e.g., condom flowers), and science projects (e.g., filling condoms with different materials and dropping them from the tops of buildings to see if Newton's theories proved to be true). David (another of Joshua's friends who had accompanied us to the movies) said with marked insight, "Well, if you can't use them for sex, you got to keep the manufacturers in business."

Two years later, in Arizona, an undergraduate education student handed me a videotape entitled *No Second Chance*, produced by Jeremiah Productions. My son, Joshua, informed me that he had seen the tape in the sex education class he had in California and again several years later in his biology class in Tempe, Arizona. I put the tape in the VCR. I sat back on my large purple velvet sofa and recoiled in horror. I was completely unprepared for the affront bombarding my sensibilities. The scenes on the videotape were frightening because the manipulation of language was done with such calculated precision. I felt as if I had stepped into a bad science fiction novel, halfway between George Orwell's *1984* and Margaret Atwood's *Handmaid's Tale*.

No Second Chance: The Wolf in Sheep's Latex
The web page for Jeremiah Productions (www.jeremiahfilms.com, 1997) reads:

> Celebrating more than 20 years in the field of video communication, Jeremiah Films continues to lead the way as an effective creator of hard-hitting, life-changing motion pictures. Through its high standards of excellence, Jeremiah Films has impacted the world with its production and distribution of intelligent, innovative, and thought-provoking films, videos, books, and music....The founder and president of Jeremiah Films is award-winning motion picture producer Patrick Matrisciana whose success has made him a much sought after radio and television talk show guest. His wife, co-founder, CEO, and creative director Caryl Matrisciana, is an internationally recognized cult expert, a bestselling author and researcher, who has coproduced many of Jeremiah Films' most successful titles....Jeremiah Films has successfully filled the void created by the national media, whose inability to consistently present the truth to the American public has become all too common. These highly informative and controversial videos have received international prominence with reviews appearing in major publications around the world. *They have been effectively used by individuals and grassroots organizations as tools to help weed out government corruption as well as promote patriotism, traditional values, and the biblical worldview of our founding fathers.* (Emphasis my own).

The web site proclaimed:

> Does the Bible have answers for hard questions on teenage sex, AIDS, treatment of the elderly, venereal disease, premarital sex, drugs, the unborn, and single parenting? Yes it does! These and other topics are challenged and discussed in these important Jeremiah Films videos.

Titles range from "The Evolution Conspiracy," "The Gay Agenda in Public Education," and "Let My Children Go" (presenting the physical and moral danger in public schools for Christian children emanating from the homosexual conspiracy in the classroom) to "Crisis in the Classroom" (exposing the radical left-wing Communist agenda at the basis of public school conspiracy in the United States) and—my personal favorite—an in-depth research report surrounding the children's novel/movie *Harry Potter and the Sorcerers's Stone* that is framed as a satanic conspiracy introducing America's children to witchcraft. I can't help but wonder, where was I when a narrow theological agenda entered into my child's classroom? Why should an esoteric Christian version of morality disguised as biology inform curricular content? How does an evangelical urge stealthily sneak into the classroom disguised as value-neutral information?

According to Mike Foster, governor of Louisiana, "Abstinence is a program that has to do with morals. Morals usually have a lot to do with religion" (Gyan, 2002:3-B). Governor Foster held a caucus at the state capitol to teach high school students about the legislative process and how to debate the issue of abstinence. Fact sheets were distributed to students, blaming the spread of sexually transmitted diseases on the removal of prayer from public schools. None of the fact sheets mentioned the removal of condoms from discussions surrounding safe sex. In this sort of climate it is very easy to understand *how*

> the Rapides Station Community Ministries, which has received more than $70,000 from the [governmentally funded] abstinence program since 1999 proclaimed publicly: "December was an excellent month for our program; we were able to focus on the Virgin birth and make it apparent that God desires sexual purity as a way of life." (Gyan, 2002:3-B)

And *why* a theatrical group traveling to high schools all around the state of Louisiana professes that sexual relations outside marriage are "offensive to God" (Gyan, 2002:3-B). And even the manner in which the Lafayette Diocese reported that they used part of the program's sexual abstinence funding to participate in prayers at abortion clinics as part of volunteer activities related to the state's sex education program (see Gyan, 2002:3-B).

Learning Lessons: An Interlude

I sat on the grass under a tree at the end of the school day with a focus group of high school students who volunteered (with parental permission) to be part of a larger research project (on the apocalypse, mutations, and science fiction). Anita, a fourteen-year-old student, stated, "America was founded by people of Christianity." In a coy voice, she rhetorically questioned, "Don't we owe it to them, to our ancestors, to keep prayer in school? Isn't it a part of our nation and our heritage?" Her friend Suzanne, braiding some blades of grass in her hands, added:

> Many stupid Democrats put their stupid ways in, because they didn't have a religion! So they let themselves rule! George Bush is doing something right bringing abstinence into schools. He is giving schools back to Americans who believe in God. Believe me, I'd rather have a president who loves God and listens to God than a president who leads us into stupid wars like Clinton and who goes against God's word. This country was first founded by the word of God! We all know that.

Benji, another student who was sitting on the grass with me, countered, "What do condoms have to do with God?" Anita said, "Everything! God tells us not to have sex, that it is a sin." Benji replied, "You say it's a sin. What about those of us who aren't Christian?" Anita replied:

> You don't have to be a "Christian." You can even be a Catholic and still believe in God and trust what he says in the Bible. Just because you don't go to church or go to a Christian or Catholic school, you can still believe in the Bible. I think that somewhere in everyone's hearts they believe in God and they would follow the Bible if given the chance. That is what our teacher said, and my parents say that too.

"You know what," Suzanne interjected, "sex is a sin, it is dirty and if you do it, you're kinda like sticking a dirty toothbrush you found on the street into your privates. Would you brush your teeth with it?" Benji started to roll his eyes and said, "How can you say sex is dirty?" Lana, Anita's seventeen-year-old sister, answered the question before Anita could begin to formulate a reply:

> Pornography diminishes sex to just an act meant for sensual pleasure, not love. By putting pornography on the computer, on TV, in magazines, and all over the place, we cheapen sex to something trivial and then we don't see its true purpose—to give life. Sex is something sacred between two people meant to give new life; it is not entertainment, although it is very easy and very tempting to think just the opposite, but also very wrong.

Benji began to rise; he reached for his backpack, not disguising his frustration. "Who cares? We should not make laws based on your morals when your 'crime' isn't hurting anyone." Suzanne tried to have the final word in the discussion: "But it does hurt America—it turns us away from God, and I am glad we are getting God back into school now....God has always belonged, that is why He's in the pledge." Benji, walking away shaking his head, said, "We put God into the pledge because of Joseph McCarthy in 1954, stupid. Something else, too, if you really do read the Bible: The Bible says be fruitful and multiply...that doesn't sound like abstinence to me." Tabitha, lying down on the grass throwing a ball up and down, was quiet during the entire conversation, staring at cloud formations. After the others left, she sat up and told me:

> I am not stupid, and so even though people say this has nothing to do with religion, it does; especially when my teacher says sex is dirty and you need to wait for marriage. I don't care about her fucking opinion because you know everyone has one. How about some information? Some of these girls, just like the girls sitting here before, think oral sex is not sex, and that anal sex is not sex, and they debate whether you are still a virgin if you are raped. But nobody is giving us information.

Post-Fordist Puritanism

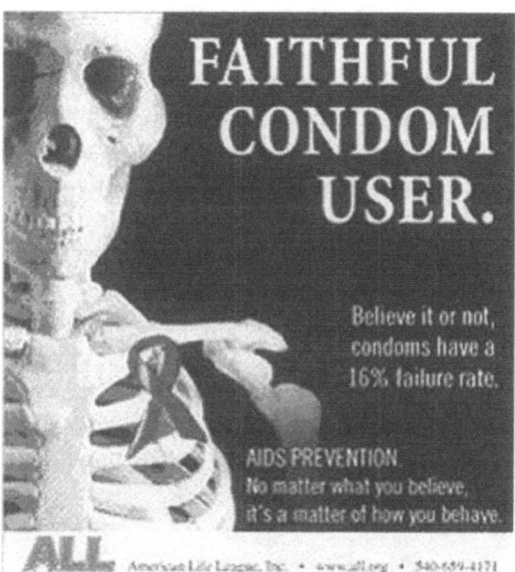

From the American Life League, www.all.org

> The infection of the mantras of the '60s affected the immune system of America. It began to accommodate the lowest and the least rather than the best and the brightest.
> —Attorney General John Ashcroft, quoted in Kintz, 1997

> The Bush administration and their ideological partners in crime would have us believe that ours was a simpler world, one in which teenagers only knew about sex what they learned from their parents and teachers. I suspect most conservatives would be horrified to discover the level of sexual knowledge most teenagers possess, would be appalled at the discussions they could overhear in any high school cafeteria. We shouldn't have to pay for their ignorance. Our nation's children should not be denied comprehensive sex education because there are those who want to believe that their kids live in a more innocent time of talks about the birds and the bees among *Brady Bunch* families. —Katherine Reilly (2002)

We are living in an age of triumphant conservative restoration. A time when the attorney general of the United States (who as a devout Pentecost does not drink, dance, or gamble) for aesthetic purposes spent $8,000 to cover up the bare breast of a statue aptly titled the Spirit of Justice (justice presumably may be blind, but she certainly is not nude). A time when U.S. officials promote policies that are diametrically opposed to what health care professionals worldwide agree are the most effective means to circumvent the continued spread of AIDS. Forty-five million more people will become infected with HIV by 2010. If condom use would be taught, 29 million of these people would never contract the virus (Lite, 2002). Selective understandings of theology position birth control as something that is universally morally wrong, irrespective of time or circumstance. The inflexibility embedded in this position is continually wrapped in a rubric of love and care (instead of in latex, which would be a lot more helpful in circumventing disease).

In modernism the mode of production may well have been related to the mode of reproduction. In post-Fordist America, however, the mode of production and the ideological intent are increasingly obscured under rubrics (ruses) of sensible (seemingly objective) policies, such as the Bush administration's resolute dogged inflexibility nationally and globally that the only sensible approach to sex education is abstinence education. As sixteen-year-old Tim commented in an exceptionally insightful manner after watching a news program on abstinence, Africa, and AIDS:

> Most people who will die of AIDS live in Africa. Do you think that anyone in the government really cares? Do you think any of the missionaries do? If Africa is depopulated we can go in there and just take the natural resources; since Africa has lots of natural resources, it can be ours along with the land. The missionaries, they get paid or get a ticket to heaven if they get more souls. It doesn't matter if the Africans are dying of starvation or of AIDS as long as they are saved; you know, like in Starvin Marvin [Starvin Marvin is a South Park cartoon character].

Tonya, a seventeen-year-old, chimed in, "We can tell people not to have sex, and they are going to listen; and when we think of Africa we are also thinking of adults." Xiomara, sixteen, added:

> In Africa, the Dark Continent, it is hot, and heat helps diseases grow. Black people live in Africa, and white people would not mourn the loss of black people no matter what they say about it—everyone knows the U.S. is racist. If Africa was empty there would be no problem exploiting their natural resources. It is all a conspiracy.

Dave added, "AIDS then spreads to communities in the United States." Seventeen-year-old Ron contributed his ideas to the conversation. "Conspiracy or not, how can you just say no to biology?"

"Because," said Risa, also seventeen. "A lot of my friends have done it and they regret it because they say it's addictive. Once you get some you want some more. It is like drugs. That's why I'm trying to wait. I don't want to become an addict." Tonya gave her a furtive look and inquired, "But it is biology, not an addiction. How can you make that comparison?" Risa remained firm in her resolve. "Because you can! Everyone knows, there have been studies done, there are doctors who talk about this. If you start taking drugs, you start having sex, or if you drink you start having sex, or if you smoke cigarettes you start having sex, and then you can't stop."

None of these responses should be surprising when placed in relation to other sheathed-stealth religious incursions into the classroom. As much as we are supposed to just say no to sex, the Scopes monkey trial is being fought again, most recently in Cobb County, Georgia. The terms of the argument were repositioned, making evolution itself a religion and creationism a scientific fact.

> Let's give our children all of the scientific information that exists. Let's not just withhold a whole body of science from them, because it doesn't fit with the religious worldview of an evolutionist...ignoring a sound scientific body. (www.cnn.com, talkbacklive, August 23, 2002)

Here in Arizona, a science teacher in a large urban public school district proclaimed proudly (during a class I taught), "I was on the textbook selection committee for science in our district. Our group elected not to choose a text with evolution in it because it was taught as fact, rather than theory." She continued to list the accomplishments of her teaching career: "I teach my students to say no to sex and the value of purity. I tell them about the importance of saving sex for after marriage. And I tell them the truth about birth control and condoms, since condoms do not work and do not prevent disease or pregnancy." The evangelical-ideological intentions are carefully reworded in a very deliberate sophisticated language game, the smoke and mirrors of obfuscation.

> To increase the appeal of this strategy for political conservatives, the New Christian Right added a "stealth" dimension in the early 1990s that entailed a softening of its often hard-edged words. The movement has replaced its explicitly religious rhetoric with the language of democracy and classical liberalism, which enables its candidates for local boards of education to hide their biblical agendas. The candidates openly associate themselves with the New Christian Right, but their mainstream rhetoric has led the public to believe that they support the values of democracy and pluralism.
> Only after the candidates become the incumbents do they unveil the often narrow meanings infusing their discourse. According to Detwiler, these candidates are "democratic in style, but not in substance" (256). He concludes that such antidemocratic presuppositions must be exposed and defeated because they conflict with the pluralistic values that most citizens hold dear. (Young, 2002: 262)

Ideological War on Condoms

David Wagner (1997), in his book *The New Temperance*, suggests that the focus on individual (immoral) behavior hides "anxieties about social class, race, and ethnicity" (6), an ideologically laden strategy "reflecting a belief in the responsibility of the state and private powers (e.g., corporations) to regulate and restrain personal behavior. The failures of self-regulation justify society's more coercive role for the presumed 'own good' of the individual" (7). Any sex except heterosexual monogamous sex (after marriage) is transformed into an addiction, with condoms seen as a form of methadone for the weak-willed. Condoms are never framed as a means of protection against disease or pregnancy, since condoms do not stop people from engaging in sexual activity. Sex, alcohol, and drugs are all conflated into a singular set of actions, all with the same outcome: the demise of (Western) civilization.

"True Love Waits" is an abstinence-based sex education program sponsored by LifeWay Christian Resources of the Southern Baptist Convention. The centerpiece of the "True Love Waits" curriculum is a signed abstinence pledge. "Think of it as a loyalty oath—except instead of saying I have never been a Communist, it says I will be a virgin till marriage," Kyle, eighteen, explained to me.

Nevertheless, 2.5 million teenagers have taken the pledge; a million of the signatures are affiliated with "True Love Waits," which has been labeled an evangelical road show for teens launched in 1993 (Williams, 2001). In California, Pennsylvania, Alabama, and many other states, schools regularly host chastity pledges and rallies on school premises during school hours. During these rituals, students often pledge "to God" that they will remain abstinent until they marry (www.plannedparenthood.org, 2002).

The web page www.truelovewaits.com for the "True Love Waits" curriculum reads:

> Believing that true love waits, I make a commitment to God, myself, my family, my friends, my future mate, and my future children to be sexually abstinent from this day until the day I enter a biblical marriage relationship.

The ideology is always expressed in the adjectives, the modifiers, and the tone. The language may well be transpositioned; the curricular packages may be slick. But the students that I interviewed, who listened to the slippage and the spaces, nailed the intentions of the program right on the (metaphorical) head. Rebecca, who recently graduated from a teacher education program in Missouri, said:

> I can't believe anyone would take seriously the lame language used by some of these programs. Who do you think they think they are targeting using hip-hop language? "Control your urgin', stay a virgin" and "Don't be a louse, wait for your spouse." To me it sounds like a cynical attempt by a bunch of white executives trying to reach black students by using slang in a pejorative racial manner but failing miserably. It is sick, really sick, even if they try to be slick; it is still sick and racist.

The Sex Respect Curriculum has been adopted by numerous school systems in the United States. It was developed by a Glenview, Illinois, organization called the Committee on the Status of Women. The group was originally founded by Phyllis Schlafly as a pro-life group that advocated for women's rights. The executive director of the Sex Respect Program, Kathleen Sullivan, publicly stated without any reservation:

> [T]he black community...[is] not going to learn to punch the time clock and to be there on time and produce a day's work if they can't even control their own emotions in the important area of sexuality. (www.pfaw.org, 2002)

This comment reinforces what Rebecca said concerning a cynical pejorative attempt to rearticulate the subject in a manner that uses identity politics (note the word "community") to reify racist stereotypes.

In another program designed for students in grades seven to nine, the textbook accompanying the audio-visual scare tactics states:

> Sociologists have found that when similar economic backgrounds ("social class") and educational levels are disregarded by couples, marriage adjustment is very difficult. Different cultural backgrounds are also hurdles too high for some couples to negotiate. (www.pfaw.org, 2002)

I doubt if a conservative Christian organization has discovered or would consider using Marxist class-based analysis. Cultural background (meaning not like American) signifies something else entirely and takes the chastity pledge to an entirely different (thinly veiled) level. I will marry only someone who comes from my background. Kali (a nineteen-year-old sophomore at a large southeastern university visiting Josh and me over break) interjected while I read out loud, "Duh, that (racism) is just totally obvious!"

Also "totally obvious" is the position taken by Dr. Robert Simonds, president of the group Citizens for Excellence in Education, based in Costa Mesa, California:

> The gay rights movement is sweeping our nation's schools....Students are told it is a normal acceptable lifestyle and that they can't criticize it because they don't know until they try it....Children have been lied to and then RECRUITED into the homosexual/lesbian lifestyle....Public school programs like "Project 10," "Children of the Rainbow" and "Project 21" are some of the many programs of homosexual/lesbianism promotion and recruitment....It's Sodom and Gomorrah all over again. Will we wait until our society is engulfed in homosexuality—lesbianism and AIDS—or stop it now? (www.pfaw.org, 2002)

Evangelical Cottage Industry

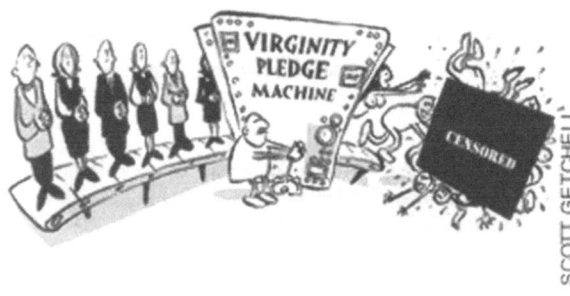

Abstinence-only programs are funded with government monies to the tune of $135 million annually, reflecting Bush's 2002 budget request for a 33 percent increase in funding annually for such programs in public schools. However, the majority of parents—81 percent—want schools to discuss the use of condoms and contraception with their children, where to go to be tested and treated for STDs, and how to sidestep unwanted sexual advances, according to a report produced by the Kaiser Family Foundation (www.kff.org, 2002).

Nine in ten sex education instructors across the country believe that students should be taught about contraceptives in school, and over one quarter report receiving explicit instructions from school boards and administrators. Today, 86 percent of school districts across the country require sex education curricula to stress abstinence (Mulrine, 2002).

Most abstinence programs created for the public schools were not designed by educators, scientists, or clinicians. On the contrary, far too many of the abstinence programs are designed by faith-based groups with a specific political agenda. The abstinence industry sprang from the loins of the anti-abortion movement.

> Some of today's abstinence leaders were part of that movement. Colleen Kelly-Mast wrote one of the earliest abstinence texts, *Sex Respect*, a workbook that has sold more than 800,000 copies. Another activist, Leslee Unruh, founded a crisis-pregnancy center in 1984, joined the Alliance of Chastity Educators and, in 1997, founded the Abstinence Clearinghouse, based in Sioux Falls, South Dakota. Marilyn Morris started in the eighties, back when the movement was explicitly faith-based and largely a volunteer effort....When her two daughters (now in their thirties) became teenagers, she vowed to tell them what no adult had told her about sex, "so (my husband and I) started talking very openly with them." When the local school found that she kept kids rapt with straight talk, they asked her to speak to eighth-grade girls. Then the church called. Then the Girl Scouts. "Suddenly," Morris says, "I was speaking everywhere." (Erard, 2002:43)

According to the Bush administration's deputy secretary of health and human services, Claude Allen, in terms of curriculum in schools "the best solutions are coming from small, faith-based and nonprofit organizations that might otherwise not be funded" (Erard, 2002:42). As an educator who is increasingly concerned about the proletarianization of the profession, I believe there may be other reasons why many abstinence programs would never be funded under other political circumstances, including the experience and qualifications of those creating the programs. I recognize that everyone knows someone who has attended school, or has attended school themselves, or has had children who have attended school—but those experiences do not necessarily create a teacher. Nevertheless, Carole Adlard received a Title V grant from the Ohio Department of Health to produce a video entitled "Why Abstinence: The Price Tag of Casual Sex" (Erard, 2002:42). Her qualifications? She is a mother of four who runs another organization in Cincinnati that both teaches abstinence and arranges adoptions.

So I guess if the program fails, since abortion is out of the question, she can continue her input: One corporation that gets you pregnant and then sells the child for you as well. There is more product diversification in her venture than if she sold or gave away condoms—she really can corner the market. She is not a health educator, a scientist, or a curriculum specialist. The above-mentioned Marilyn Morris's qualification as a curriculum designer is that she became pregnant before marriage (okay, I admit she also seems to do a very good imitation of Marlon Brando in *On the Waterfront*). "I coulda had everything," she laments. "I coulda had tennis, I coulda had college, I coulda had a wonderful wedding, I coulda had a family...I just could have had everything" (Erard, 2002:43).

Deputy Secretary Claude Allen's firm commitment to abstinence programs is because they "instill values as well as provide information" (Erard, 2002:42).

Whose values? But what sort of information is being spread? In viewing the *No Second Chance* video, the only information I see is disingenuous disinformation. In listening to many other programs and reviewing the curriculums, the misinformation is glaring and dangerous. Listen to what one eighteen-year-old thought:

> Technically, if you don't have intercourse involving a penis and a vagina, you are a virgin. The hymen in the female will break. However, nothing physically changes about the guy, and it is said he lost his virginity, making it more of a symbolic thing, if that makes sense. So oral and anal sex don't technically take physical virginity away, but they take mental virginity away, which is what the guy loses in intercourse. Does that make sense?

A student teacher raised with "good family values" (a self-description) says:

> What if you are raped? Yes, you can still be considered a virgin. Virginity is not something that can be taken from you; it is something that you give. Also, when you give your virginity, you give a part of your heart, something which also cannot be taken from you.

These conversations seem absurd in 2005, but they proliferate because of the lack of information on sexuality.

> In 1998, a survey of freshmen and sophomores at Southern colleges showed "a quarter considered anal intercourse as abstinence and more than a third surveyed did

not consider oral sex to be sex." The figure rose when no one involved had an orgasm. Numbers were similar for masturbation with another person. If you think this is surprising, hold on to your hat: a 1999 survey disclosed that nearly a third of health educators believe that oral sex constitutes abstinence. The tragedy here is manifestly self-evident: you can still contract sexually transmitted diseases, including syphilis, chlamydia, gonorrhea, and herpes through unprotected oral sex. Likewise, unprotected anal sex is highly conducive to HIV transmission. But there's also a delicious irony: by insisting on abstinence, the "just say no" culture of Christian conservatism is producing a generation of youth who've embraced sexual acts that not only are traditionally considered "deviant"—but are illegal in 18 states. This is no mean feat for a political movement that is doing its damnedest to inculcate, if not mandate, a standard of "normal" and "responsible" sexual behavior in its young people...there's a startling connection between the right wing's tenacious definition of "real sex" as heterosexual and reproductive (and permissible only within the confines of marriage) and the new, widespread belief that anal and oral sex fall squarely outside the definition of "sex."(Bronski, 2001)

The *No Second Chance* video is but one example of the extent and pervasiveness of this bizarre, dangerous neo-medievalism—which is nothing short of "educational malpractice" (Bronski, 2001). Sure, creationism is not a science, and the earth may well be flat, and Jesus may be coming back at any moment, but my son does not risk dying through falling off the earth from deliberately constructed falsehoods, such as those seen in the video *No Second Chance*.

The setting is a (contrived) classroom, unlike any classroom I have ever encountered. The rows are neat, the students all scrubbed, starched, and attentive. A student asks, "What if I want to have sex before I get married?" The teacher (school nurse/authority figure) replies, "Well, I guess you just have to be prepared to die. And you'll probably take your spouse and one or more of your children with you." Further, the figure of authority explains ridiculous unfounded concepts, such as "secondary virginity."

In another scene, in which a gun is pointed directly at the camera, "condom use is depicted as a game of Russian roulette." The same metaphor is stated explicitly in the workbook for another abstinence curriculum entitled "Choosing the Best": "When you use a condom, it is like playing Russian roulette. There is a greater risk of a condom failure than the bullet being in the chamber" (www.siecus.org).

The scare tactics etched into abstinence-based curriculums work "to make condoms seem like the culprit in the AIDS pandemic, rather than a means of reducing one's risk during intercourse. Safe sex is described as a myth, and condoms as a false hope" (www.siecus.org, 2002). Typical with abstinence-based curricular approaches are false assertions surrounding the failure rate of condoms, backed up with data based on a variety of statistical and methodological fallacies, in addition to a wide array of hyperbolic histrionic proclamations. In Choosing the Best, condoms are described as extremely complicated to use, requiring a minimum of ten steps, including:

> inspecting the condom for holes and leaks before using, putting on the condom as you begin foreplay, using proper lubricants, leaving an air space, using spermicide, careful removal of the condom, immediate washing of the genital areas with both soap and water and either rubbing alcohol or dilute solutions of Lysol®. The final step mentioned, washing the genital areas, has no relationship to condom use and applying rubbing alcohol or Lysol® to the genitals could be extremely damaging. (www.siecus.org, 2002)

This description is followed by the claim that "condoms have a 20 percent failure rate and that over a five-year period, 67 out of 100 individuals using a condom would be infected...If this process continues [Choosing the Best states] for 20 years, 99% of our original group of 100 would be infected" (www.siecus.org, 2002). The authors of this claim are forgetting or neglecting the statistical fact that probability is not cumulative.

In the *No Second Chance* video, the teacher explains in all seriousness to the captive room of Stepford children, "The next time that somebody wants you to go to bed with them, with or without a condom, then just picture that...it's not just you and him or you and her: It's that you're packing along a loaded revolver with you when you go." Giving new meaning to Mae West's old line: "Is that a pistol in your pocket or are you happy to see me?"

An Ending and a Parable

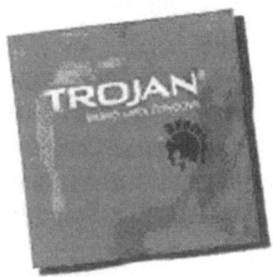

> I would be laughing if it weren't so sad. Of course, abstinence should be taught, even encouraged. But to be the sole method of birth control—you've got to be kidding! —Parent of a fifteen-year-old

> Sex ed programs that teach abstinence—that's fine. Sex ed classes that teach *only* abstinence—*no way*! School ought to be a place where full, accurate, nonbiased FACTS are taught. Children and teens need to learn the basics of reproductive anatomy and the reproductive process, including birth control options, how they work, *and* how they fail...to withhold information about contraceptives is a gross disservice to our kids. I thought America kept religion and schooling separate; the "wait-until-marriage" idea is a religious one based on the idea that sex is sinful—I am disgusted that political leaders are allowing educational decisions to be determined by the religious conservatives. Teach facts in school, please, and do not withhold information from teens that they may need to know. —Parent of a twelve-year-old

I found the following comment on the floor along with other discarded parts of the transcripts I collected for this chapter. "Condoms are like a Trojan horse (perhaps that is why one condom company is named Trojan). You think you are protected but you are not." I do not know who said it. But it seems to be an appropriate sentence encompassing all sides of this debate (which ought not be a debate at all). A practice engendered by an increasingly racist, homophobic, theological curriculum in the public schools does nothing to educate students about something that has direct consequences on their lives. Who would think that one little latex package could stir up such deeply rooted sensations?

A mother of three children ages twelve, fifteen, and seventeen states:

> We are hiding our heads in the sand if we think abstinence is the way to go. Teenagers deserve to be told all the truth. They live in a world very different from Bush and the other policy makers, who seem to dwell in a very naive place. What a travesty this is going to be. Today we have diseases that kill. Yes, I want my children to wait until marriage, but as a person who spent twenty years in health care, I have seen firsthand what ignorance does. I have had twelve-year-old girls tell me they thought they were pregnant, because they did not understand the mechanics of sex—or the outcome of intercourse. While abstinence is the only way to prevent—100 percent—sexually transmitted diseases and unwanted pregnancy, we all know that this is shortsighted and actually really the sickest policy I have ever heard of. I think that our children deserve respect: They do grow up! Or, at least I hope they do.

Rebecca is about to embark on her teaching career this year. She says:

> It worries me that kids don't know what a clitoris is (just like on *South Park*) and that eighteen-year-olds might find the same uses for condoms as your son and his friends did when they were in middle school. These programs promote nothing but ignorance. There will be lasting consequences for this country, not to say worldwide as well. It is getting very weird here.

In America in 2005 we can cover up a cold stone statue to shield the eyes of the attorney general, but we cannot shield our children from pregnancy and disease by explaining the use of a little latex cover.

Bibliography

Acland, R. (1994). *Youth, murder, spectacle*. Boulder, CO: Westview Press.

Alcoff, L. (1995). Mestizo identity. In N. Zack (Ed.), *American mixed race: The culture of microdiversity*. Lanham, MD: Rowman and Littlefield.

American Life League (2002). *Pro-life without exception, without compromise, without apology*. Available from: www.all.org.

Anagnost, A. (2000). Scenes of misrecognition: Maternal citizenship in the age of transnational adoption. *Positions, 8*(2): 389–421.

Angrosino, M. (2002). Civil religion redux. *Anthropological Quarterly, 75* (2): 239–267. Available from http://muse.jhu.edu/journals/anthropological_quarterly/v075/75.2angrosino.html.

Anijar, K. (1998). Childhood and caring: A capitalist taxonomy of the mar(x)et place. In M. Hauser and J. Jipson (Eds.), *Intersections/feminisms/early childhoods*. New York: Peter Lang.

Anijar, K., and Casey, C. (1997). Adolescent as curriculum theorist. *Journal for a Just and Caring Education, 3*(4): 381–399.

Apple, M. (2000a). *Official knowledge*. 2nd edition. New York: Routledge.

———. (2000b). Can critical pedagogies interrupt rightist policies? *Educational Theory, 50*(2): 229–254.

———. (1996). *Cultural politics and education*. New York: Teachers College Press.

Berlant, L. G. (1997). *The queen of America goes to Washington City: Essays on sex and citizenship*. Durham, NC: Duke University Press.

———. (1991). *The anatomy of national fantasy: Hawthorne, utopia, and everyday life*. Chicago: University of Chicago Press.

Berliner, D. C. (1997). Educational psychology meets the Christian right: Differing view of children, schooling, teaching, and learning. *Teachers College Record, 98*(3): 381–416.

Bronski, M. (2001). Christian sex outlaws. *The Worcester Phoenix,* 8–15 February. Available from: *www.worcesterphoenix.com/archive/features/01/02/08/ sex_outlaw.html*.

Broughton, J. (1996). The bomb's eye view. In S. Aronowitz, B. Martinson, and S. Mesner (Eds.), *Techno science and cyber culture*. New York: Routledge.

CNN (2002). Talk back: Live transcript from August 23, 2002. Available from: *www.cnn.com*.

Cook, B. (1993). *Choosing the best*. Atlanta, GA: Choosing the Best Publications.

D'Emilio, J. (1996). Capitalism and gay identity. In D. Morton (Ed.), *The material queer*. Boulder, CO: Westview Press.

Erard, M. (2002). Virgins, Inc. *Rolling Stone,* 25 April, 41–44.

Falla, J. (2001). Disorderly consumption and capitalism: The privilege of sex addiction. *College Literature, 28*(1): 46–64.

Foucault, M. (1978). *The history of sexuality, Volume I: An introduction.* Trans. Robert Hurley. New York: Vintage Press.

Giroux, H. (2001). Pedagogy of the depressed: Beyond the new politics of cynicism. *College Literature, 28*(3): 1–33.

———. (1995). White panic. In C. Berlet (Ed.), *Eyes right: Challenging the right-wing backlash*. Boston: South End Press.

———. (1992). *Border crossings: Cultural workers and the politics of education*. New York: Routledge.

Gyan, J. (2002). ACLU sues state over abstinence program: Lawsuit says tax dollars used to promote religion. *Baton Rouge State-Times/Morning Advocate*, 11 May, Sec. 3-B.

Jeremiah Films (1997). Available from: *www.jeremiahfilms.com*.

Kaiser Family Foundation (2002). Available from: *www.kff.org*.

Keating, A. (1995). Interrogating "whiteness," (de)constructing race. *College English, 57(*8): 901–918.

Kincheloe, J. (2000). Introducton in Anijar, K., *Teaching towards the 24th century: The social curriculum of Star Trek*. New York: Routledge.

———. (1999). The struggle to define and reinvent whiteness: a pedagogical analysis. *College Literature, 26*(3): 162–190.

———. (1995). *Toil and trouble: Good work, smart workers, and the integration of academic and vocational education*. New York: Peter Lang.

Kincheloe, J., and S. Steinberg (1997). *Changing multiculturalism*. London: Open University Press.

Kincheloe, J., S. Steinberg, N. Rodriguez, and R. Chennault (Eds.). (1998). *White reign: Deploying whiteness in America*. New York: St. Martin's Press.

Kintz, L. (1997). *Between Jesus and the market*. Durham, NC: Duke University Press.

Lite, J. (2002). Morality and AIDS. *Nation, 275*(5): 5–7.

Mackler. C. (August–September 1999). Sex ed: How do we score? *Ms. Magazine* online. Available from: *www.msmagazine.com*.

Mulrine, A. (2002). Risky business. *U.S. News & World Report, 132*(18): 42–50.

People for the American Way (2002). *Teaching fear: The religious right's campaign against sexuality education* (originally published 1996). www.pfaw.org.

Planned Parenthood (2002). *Abstinence-only education: Why first amendment supporters should oppose it.* Available from: www.plannedparenthoodnj.org/library/files/28_2002102313.pdf

Readings, B. (1996). *The university in ruins.* Cambridge, MA: Harvard University Press.

Reilly, K. (2002, February 21). Abstinence programs encourage deadly silence. *The Daily Princetonian.* Princeton, NJ: Princeton University.

Sexuality Information and Educational Council of the United States (2002). Available from: www.siecus.org.

Wagner, D. (1997). *The new temperance.* Boulder, CO: Westview Press.

Williams, Z. (2001). Faith, hope, and chastity. *The Guardian,* 20 October. Available from: www.guardian/uk.com.

Young, J. (2002). Standing on the premises of God: The Christian right's fight to redefine America's public schools. *Quarterly Journal of Speech, 88*(2): 262–264.

Zizek, S. (1993). *Tarrying with the negative: Kant, Hegel, and the critique of ideology.* Durham, NC: Duke University Press.

• CHAPTER TWO •

When Condoms Go Bad:
From Safe Sex to Five Microns to *Killer Condom*

Thuy DaoJensen

And when something is about masculinity, it is not always "about men."
—Eve Kosofsky Sedgwick

During the late 1980s and early 1990s, increased medical research on the AIDS epidemic led to awareness campaigns in the United States that promoted the use of condoms as a "safe sex" strategy that could lower the risk of transmitting the AIDS virus during sexual activity. Condoms became synonymous with "safe sex" and were distributed free of charge in many public places, such as family planning clinics and college campuses. But with the widespread distribution of condoms, religious groups such as Christian evangelicals and Catholics decried the cultural depravity and immorality associated with condoms and sexual promiscuity outside the context of marriage.

Developed by members of the gay community and AIDS activists, the safe sex programs that promoted condoms viewed the messages of sexual abstinence and monogamy from religious groups to be homophobic. Once the decreasing rate of AIDS transmission in the gay community was documented, professional health educators in the heterosexual community began to legitimize and appropriate a more comprehensive sex education that included a safe-sex message of condoms for the heterosexual population. Given the extensive medical research on sexual behavior and diseases conducted by health professionals around the country, how did the discourse of religious morality come to influence the perception of condoms?

Sociologist Janice Irvine (2002) writes that "an important way to foster morality in contemporary American culture is through the establishment of expertise" (p.115). By creating their own medical research institutes such as Family Research Council and the Medical Institute for Sexual Health, religious organizations could claim the authority of scientific knowledge and medical expertise in their crusade against a more comprehensive sex education that advocated condoms. The dubious nature of the medical research and findings of these institutions obscured the ideological differences even as it helped to engineer a backlash against the safe sex campaigns of condom usage.

A report called "Condom Roulette" released by the conservative Family Research Council (1992) argued that condoms had holes that measured five microns. Apparently, using a condom was analogous to a deadly game of putting a spinning gun barrel to one's head with a finger on the trigger. Based on studies of latex gloves that generalized those findings to latex condoms, the report argued that these holes were impenetrable for sperm to pass through, yet the HIV virus measuring 0.1 to 0.3 microns could pass. While researchers at the Centers for Disease Control in Atlanta determined the findings to be deceptive and confusing by comparing latex gloves and condoms, religious groups could now claim that there were life-threatening risks involved with sexual behavior, generating suspicion of condoms as a "safe sex" method in the prevention of AIDS.

Christian Right in the Curriculum
By the beginning of the twenty-first century, religious groups used this medical expertise to establish a secular sex education curriculum to promote an abstinence-only message in American public schools. The grass-roots mobilization of the gay community in promoting condoms as safe sex was replaced by data from the conservative research institutes that concluded condoms had a failure rate ranging from 15 to 50 percent.

To frame the effectiveness of condoms in preventing pregnancy and STD transmission in terms of failure rates is a form of gross misrepresentation that works to instill fear in young adults, as these failure rates are used to justify the abstinence-only messages that "condoms fail." As an educational researcher, I have witnessed abstinence-only instructors from religiously affiliated organizations going into public schools, drawing from the misleading type of research put out by Family Research Council. They downplay the safe-sex message of condoms by relating anecdotes of doctors who would not risk their own lives by wearing gloves made of the same material as latex condoms during surgery. At the end of the story, the rhetorical question posed to students is, "If doctors won't even risk their lives over latex, would you?"

Abstinence-only educators assert that the only method that carries a 100 percent success rate is total abstinence from premarital sexual activity, followed by monogamy. According to abstinence-only educators, the grave conclusion is that there is no such thing as "safe sex."

While the concern is that the abstinence-only programs are preventing young adults from obtaining information about condoms as prophylaxis, there needs to be an exploration of the cultural shift occurring in conceptualizing the usage of condoms as a safe sex method to claims by conservative groups that holes in condoms make sexual activity a dangerous and life-threatening experience that could lead to contracting the HIV virus and inevitable death. As the cultural theorist Stuart Hall wrote, "AIDS is the site at which the advance of sexual politics is being rolled back. It's a site at which not only people will die, but desire and pleasure will also die if certain metaphors do not survive, or survive in the wrong way" (1992, p. 285). Indeed, the metaphor of safe sex and condoms may have dissipated as the fear of five microns dilutes the campaign of AIDS education. In this chapter, I explore how the socially constructed symbolic meanings of condoms within the safe/dangerous binary reflecting underlying cultural tensions and ambivalence in contradictory messages about condoms and sexuality are portrayed in the German cult film *Killer Condom: The Rubber That Rubs You Out*.

Killer Condom: **The Movie**

As a German film with English subtitles, *Kondom des Grauens* or *Killer Condom* (1997) manages to horrify as well as entertain viewers with images of a carnivorous condom with protruding fangs. Giving new meaning to the idea of sexual protection, director Martin Walz's film manages to intertwine the competing narratives of the acceptance of homosexuality as a lifestyle choice against the homophobic religious zealots whose quest to rid New York City of them results in the creation of a genetically altered condom crossed with a piranha. Science and religion have come together to reveal the nagging doubt that condoms may not offer much in terms of "safe sex" practices.

As narrated by the protagonist, Luigi Macaroni, New York City is a "playground for perverts," replete with trope imagery of illicit adult stores and pornography, signifiers that predate Mayor Giuliani's policies to sanitize the sex industry in Times Square. Macaroni is an openly gay city detective of Italian ethnicity, called in to investigate the several male castrations at Hotel Quickie, a seedy hotel known for its gay clientele and prostitution. As part of the city's safe sex campaign, condoms (rubbers) are placed on the bedside table in every hotel room. Suspiciously, none of them are individually wrapped, as they are cheaper to acquire in bulk.

The opening scene shows a male school administrator who has lured a reluctant, weeping teenage girl into the hotel for sexual favors so that she can pass her exams. When the *Killer Condom* has bitten off the school administrator's genitalia and that of other men at Hotel Quickie, the police assume that the girl and other female prostitutes are the culprits behind the onslaught of castrations. The girl's trauma leads the police to contact her parents, warning them that their daughter has been corrupted by the danger in the city while suggesting that they return to their safe and simple lifestyle back in Farmville, Oklahoma.

During an investigation of Hotel Quickie, Macaroni indulges in his desires when he meets a young gay male prostitute named Billy. Macaroni, in spite of his name, is a well-endowed man, measuring 32 centimeters. It is during this encounter that the Killer Condom tries unsuccessfully to castrate his penis but manages to remove his right testicle. Feeling fortunate to have escaped penis castration, Macaroni is determined to stop the bloodshed, even as his colleagues at the police station joke and laugh in disbelief at the idea of a "crazed contraceptive" or "*killer condom.*"

Macaroni's relief that the Killer Condom has not removed his penis underscores deep cultural anxieties over castration, male sexual performance, and masculinity. The condom may provide protection from disease and serve as a method of contraception, but the irony is that male castration itself has also served as form of contraception in the past. In Macaroni's case, using a condom for contraceptive purposes is superfluous, since he is gay. However, the meaning of male castration and what it entails has not remained static, but rather has changed throughout history.

Gary Taylor (2002) writes that in ancient times, castration focused on removing the male testicles, not the penis. The eunuch was a castrated male, an artificially sterilized male who could still perform sexually but was unable to impregnate a woman. Taylor credits Sigmund Freud's controversial psychoanalytic theory of castration anxiety with the evolving obsession toward penis castration, yet in Taylor's analysis, Freud was "mistaken about history and anatomy." Freud's misplaced understanding of castration raises the question: What qualifies as masculinity in our culture? While male genitalia seem to be of great importance, is masculinity the ability to perform sexually, or is it related to the number of offspring a male produces?

Assuming that most men would choose to use a condom over the surgical alternative of testicle amputation, the fear of castration may just as well apply to condoms that supposedly protect the penis. Some men may find the condom emasculating; they are opposed to using one either because it disrupts the spontaneity of foreplay or it decreases male pleasure. In any of these cases, the sexual acts could be either homosexual or heterosexual, since the threat of castration is tacitly embedded in the social construction of masculinity.

In terms of masculinity and male genitalia, Taylor argues that the "historical shift from the primacy of the scrotum to the primacy of the penis" represents a cultural shift in sexual behaviors from patrilineal reproduction to the penis as the "locus of male pleasure" (p. 108). In the realm of male sexual pleasure, sexual activity need not be conceptually limited to heterosexual acts or procreative purposes only. While the use of condoms has further complicated the perception of male pleasure in secular discourse, distinct positions have also emanated from religious discourse toward the male body. "Official Christianity has remained the chief site of resistance to the emergent regime of penises and pleasure; even now fundamentalist Christians continue to campaign against a proliferation of behaviors that they characterize as 'perversions.'" (Taylor, 2002, p.108). The articulation of sexual pleasure as perversion imposes a certain gender hierarchy within a symbolic framework.

The denouncing of sexual pleasure as base and perverted is a common narrative that continues in modern-day sexual rhetoric, most notably in *Killer Condom*. In addition to investigating the Killer Condom, Detective Macaroni struggles with his well-meaning colleagues who try to convince him to abandon his gay lifestyle for a heterosexual one. The other officers are wary and skeptical of a Killer Condom presence, preferring to blame the male prostitute Billy for Macaroni's castration. Eventually Macaroni is vindicated by the Killer Condom's castration of a Republican presidential candidate at the upscale Waldorf-Astoria Hotel.

Dick McGouvern's campaign speeches, like those of many other presidential candidates, nostalgically beckon for American politics to "regain its values and belief in God." Calling for a society that needs to be healed in order to make the country strong once more, he urges the people to unite with him for a "clean America" that is free of "scandals, drugs, and perversity." At the upscale hotel, Killer Condom attacks McGouvern as he relaxes in his bathtub while his mistress looks on with horror and disbelief. The following day's newspaper headlines dub the candidate "Dickless Dick," infuriating and embarrassing McGouvern's staff, as they know that the American people will never vote for a man *sans penis*, the symbolic equivalent of masculinity, leadership, and virility. The castration of a presidential candidate by the Killer Condom can be viewed as an emasculating process in which not only his reproductive organs are removed but also any aspirations he had in fulfilling a world leadership position as the American president.

Granted, the portrayal of American attitudes is somewhat distorted through the lens of German filmmakers, yet it confronts contradictory values of masculinity and sexuality in the way Americans view presidential candidates. The sexual prowess of candidate Bill Clinton may have been a non-issue in getting elected, and to some extent even his sexual indiscretions hardly affected his job approval ratings. Yet the idea of an overactive libido outside of marriage prompts feelings of outrage and disgust for some Americans. Would the American public knowingly accept a president who reveals himself to be a castrated male?

The climactic ending of *Killer Condom* has Luigi being led back to the church next to the city hospital where so many castrated victims of the Killer Condom are treated. At the church, he discovers that the creator of the Killer Condom is a former Soviet scientist kidnapped and being held against his will in a scientific laboratory below the church by a female doctor, Dr. Riffleson. Conflating Cold War anxieties, Christian morality, and anti-feminist backlash, Dr. Riffleson is an unmarried woman who purports to be a Christian feminist. She is a caricature of spinster bitterness, intent on performing "God's work" by castigating and castrating the gay male community for engaging in sexual activity that transgresses the religious principle of procreation. Ironically, gay men remain central to the *Killer Condom* narrative, as the religious zealots seem uninterested in lesbians and heterosexual women, failing to do "God's work" by creating a deadly female condom.

To frame feminists as emasculating men is nothing new; Freud's theory of females who resist male domination through pathological fantasies of castrating men have conflated patriarchal ideology and myth-making to the point of unquestioned fact. Like the teen horror films that portray the inevitable murder of sexually active youth as a form of entertainment, *Killer Condom* seems to fit this genre. While the film's third-rate special effects will leave many viewers unsatisfied, the notion of a "Killer Condom" signifies the many competing discourses concerning sexual activity in our culture, imbuing comic relief while reflecting tensions and anxiety over sexual activity for procreation versus merely for pleasure. In the post-safe-sex era, is there a space for dialogue about condoms that moves beyond the safe/dangerous binary?

Bibliography

Butler, J. (1990). *Gender trouble*. New York: Routledge.

———. (1995). Melancholy gender/Refused identification. In M. Berger, B. Wallis, & S. Watson (Eds.), *Constructing masculinity* (pp. 21–36). New York: Routledge.

Dietrich, R., Reichebner, H., & Walz, M. (Director). (1997). *Killer condom: The rubber that rubs you out* [Motion picture]. Germany: Troma Entertainment, Inc.

Family Research Council (1992). "Condom Roulette." *In Focus*, May 1992: 1–4.

Hall, S. (1992). Cultural studies and its theoretical legacies. In L. Grossberg, C. Nelson, & P. Treichler (Eds.), *Cultural Studies* (pp. 277–294). London: Routledge.

Irvine, J. (1990). *Disorders of desire*. Philadelphia: Temple University Press.

———. (2002). *Talk about sex: The battles over sex education in the United States*. Berkeley: University of California Press.

Sedgwick, E. K. (1995). "Gosh, Boy George, you must be awfully secure in your masculinity!" In M. Berger, B. Wallis, & S. Watson (Eds.), *Constructing masculinity* (pp. 11–20). New York: Routledge.

Taylor, G. (2002). *Castration: An abbreviated history of western manhood*. New York: Routledge.

• CHAPTER THREE •

Queer Eye on the Straight Guy's Condoms

Jessamyn Neuhaus

Yes, it perpetuates certain stereotypes about the gender behavior of both straight and gay men. Yes, it glorifies consumerism, elitism, a deeply materialistic worldview, and obsessive attention to one's "image." Yes, it's one of the most successful of the "reality TV" shows—a media trend that I abhor. That being said, I also believe that *Queer Eye for the Straight Guy* is an important and hopeful sign in mainstream popular culture that a critical mass of people in the United States accept and, indeed, cheerfully rejoice in the fact that some of us are queer. And the brief but highly significant appearance of a package of condoms on the first episode of the second season of *Queer Eye for the Straight Guy* demonstrates this fact.

The premise of *Queer Eye for the Straight Guy* (*QE*) is similar to that of other "makeover" shows. In each episode, five lifestyle experts—Ted Allen (food and wine), Kyan Douglas (grooming), Thom Filicia (interior design), Jai Rodriguez (culture), and Carson Kressley (fashion)—transform a male slob in need of home decorating, cooking instruction, clothes shopping, and hair styling into a well-coifed, culturally sophisticated man. The catch? The makeover team is gay and the slob-turned-fabulous is straight. Or rather, the straight man becomes a newly born "metrosexual"—a term made mainstream almost entirely due to the influence of this show. First used by British author and cultural commentator Mark Simpson, a metrosexual is a (usually heterosexual) man who is unabashedly stylish, trend-conscious, and sensitive to the home decorating needs of his mate.[1] *QE* premiered in July 2003 on the NBC-owned Bravo Network and enjoyed instant success, averaging 2.5 million viewers by September. The stars of the show soon made guest appearances on *The Tonight Show* and *Oprah Winfrey*, and today fans of the show maintain numerous web sites and purchase thousands of *QE* books, calendars, and CDs.

NBC executives almost immediately planned for a second season of *QE* and on December 9, 2003, the first episode of Season Two aired. Entitled "An Officer and a Gentleman," this episode features the Fab Five tackling the apartment and appearance of Ross M., former Marine and new cohabitant of girlfriend Teresa, who is eager for Ross to ditch the boring khakis and sloppy bachelor pad decor. The team begins, as they do every episode, by good-naturedly rifling through the straight subject's cupboards and closets, freely criticizing his taste in cookware and clothes and his lack of a skin care regimen. In ransacking Ross's dresser drawers, Thom Filicia happens across two or three single packages of condoms. He says, "So now you and Teresa are living in sin? A nice wholesome Marine like yourself?" Giggling sheepishly, Ross replies, "You're just going to go through everything, aren't you?" Thom answers mockingly, "I just want to find out all your secrets."

The very next scene plays off the preceding condom references. Carson Kressley holds up what looks like a long, flat, skinny sleeping bag and asks, "What is this?" Ross answers, "That's called my surf sock...to cover my stick." Eyebrows raised, innuendo in voice, Carson says, "Really!" And in the third and final reference to the condoms, Thom says to Teresa, "If we design this as a sensual place, you'll finally be able to get to use these!" She too giggles sheepishly and mumbles, "Oh, we don't use those." Thom, with his arm around her shoulder, mock-scolds, "You don't use them? Gosh, you use the rhythm method or something?"

The tone and nature of these dialogues are absolutely typical of the show. This first segment of each episode always features rapid, cattily hilarious, and often sexually suggestive banter. The stars of *QE* strike an important balance in these initial contacts with the straight subject—and with their audience. The *QE* team members' primary function is to serve as highly qualified experts in each of their respective fields, and the vast majority of their recorded dialogue is advice and explanation about cooking, decorating, and clothing. But they are also completely comfortable acknowledging their shared homosexual identity with flirty remarks to the straight subject and affectionate touching and slang terms with each other. Snaps for that! Significantly, the stars of *QE* are playfully and wittily confronting and rejecting a long-standing excuse for homophobia: the myth that gay men are always wildly attracted to straight men and are unable to control their sexual overtures toward straight men. The *QE* team laughs in the face of that tired old story. So do the straight men, who invariably play along with the joke and recognize this flirty behavior as simply that: a joke among men comfortable with their different sexual object choices.

The *QE* team's main mission, in fact, is to make the straight guy more attractive to his female mate or potential mate. In episode after episode, the *QE* team confers with the female spouse or girlfriend, who pleads with the Fab Five to make her straight guy more attentive to his personal appearance, more aware of the joys of shopping for home furnishings, more open to style and culture, and more attuned to the importance of cleaning up and sharing one's space, life, and recreation with a woman. In "An Officer and a Gentleman," for example, Thom remakes the slovenly bachelor pad into a grown-up space where Teresa feels comfortable too. Jai gives Ross dancing lessons and tickets to the hottest salsa club in town—what woman doesn't want to be taken out dancing by her significant other? Far from remaking straight guys into gay guys, the stars of *QE* make straight guys into *better* straight guys. "All things just keep getting better," trills the refrain for the show's theme song.[2]

The brief appearance of condoms on episode #114 demonstrates how *Queer Eye for the Straight Guy* accepts, even humorously celebrates, sexual difference and how the stars play with their roles as gay authorities. The initial discovery of the condoms, for example, is immediately seized upon as a topic for poking gentle fun at heterosexuality. First Thom mocks the concept of a "nice, wholesome Marine" by pointing out the condoms. Then, sweetly dismissing Ross's embarrassment, Thom remarks he's just discovering Ross's secrets. The "secret" here is that straight Marines have sex and use condoms—*not* that the stylish home decorator is gay. Thom, with his discovery of the condoms, has the power to comment on, even mock, the sexual behavior of the heterosexual man. What a reversal of the usual power dynamic, where gay men are the vulnerable ones! With just a few good-humored jibes, Thom neatly upends the assumption that gay men are the ones with a secret and that gay male sexual practices are suspect and open to derision by straight men.

One of the most pleasurable parts of watching *Queer Eye for the Straight Guy* is seeing precisely this kind of reversal. Here, it is queer men who are the experts, who are the voice of authority, and who have the power, indeed the responsibility, to comment on the lives of heterosexuals. Of course, the fact that this power is limited to stereotypically "gay" areas of expertise is troubling, as is the stark difference between the Fab Five's power within the confines of a reality TV show and the struggle for gay and lesbian civil rights in the real world. Yet we must also acknowledge that it can be deeply satisfying to see heterosexual men and women listen closely and attentively to the words of gay men and acknowledge their authority.[3] And as this initial exchange about condoms shows, the *QE* team's comments are not always limited to "lifestyle" issues such as soufflé recipes and hair-styling product: Thom comments on Ross's heterosexual sexual behavior. After listening to far too many straight politicians comment on the sexual behavior of homosexuals, I find Thom's remarks a welcome relief.

Thom again comments on heterosexual sexual practices when Teresa says, "Oh, we don't use those." Thom's gasp of disbelief, although meant humorously, has several layers of meaning here. First, when he replies, "Gosh, you use the rhythm method or something?" he ridicules both the heterosexual need for contraception and the cavalier way many heterosexuals fail to use contraception. His arm around her shoulder shows that he's only teasing, but Thom's remark demonstrates, again, the reversal of power: the gay man editorializing on the straight person's sexual practices.

Secondly, and much more subtly, Thom's reaction is a comment on the signification of condoms in gay and straight sexual practices. Obviously, for a gay man, using condoms has nothing to do with contraception: the condom's only function is to prevent sexually transmitted diseases. Interestingly, providing protection against STDs among heterosexuals is what facilitated the condom's transition from black market novelty to mainstream acceptability in the United States. During World War II, widespread concern in the top levels of the United States military about venereal disease among the enlisted men led government policy makers to condone the distribution of condoms to the troops. Officials even urged soldiers to use condoms when on "R&R." Widespread sale of condoms to the general public soon followed.[4]

But perhaps the most significant way that Americans have utilized condoms to prevent disease occurred with the onset of the AIDS epidemic in the 1980s, when millions of gay men were extraordinarily quick to incorporate the use of condoms into their sexual practices to prevent the spread of HIV. Teresa is in a committed, presumably monogamous relationship, apparently unconcerned about venereal disease and probably using another form of birth control. Thom's reaction is a funny but compelling reminder that condoms serve another function in addition to birth control—and that this function had and continues to have a profound impact on the lives of gay men. There is no "rhythm method" that will prevent the transmission of HIV and other STDs, a fact that Teresa (and all straight, sexually active people) should bear in mind.

Finally, Carson's raised eyebrow in response to the "cover my stick" remark is instructive. The "stick" and the surfboard cover clearly evoke a penis and a condom. The humor in the exchange is based on the simple fact that Carson, as a gay man, is sexually attracted to other gay men (and their penises)—and that Ross knows this and the viewer know this. Similar jokes based on the Fab Five's sexual object choices appear regularly on the show.

This kind of humor is perhaps rather puerile, but I find it immensely hopeful. Hopeful because when I see these exchanges, I'm seeing gay and straight men joking together about sexuality, using humor to disarm what has far too often been an excuse for intimidation, abuse, and violence. No matter that it's contained on the totally artificial environment of a reality TV show: *Queer Eye for the Straight Guy* simply assumes that its viewers and its subjects will accept its stars' queerness.

From the title itself to the fact that these men unashamedly embrace stereotypically "gay" occupations to sexually suggestive encounters such as the condom remarks in the episode "An Officer and a Gentlemen," the producers and stars of the show never for a moment doubt that America is more than ready to discard homophobia like last season's shoes. And nowhere is that more evident than in the stars' ability to poke fun at the stereotype of the oversexed homosexual. As columnist Bruce Steele wrote for *The Advocate*: "They even effortlessly refute the canard of the predatory gay man hankering for some straight booty: They slap and tickle, and everyone gets the joke. Flirting is just good fun, not a sexual assault. In a way that must drive Scalia crazy, the Fab 5 are both aggressively sexual and nonthreatening."[5]

The "canard of the predatory gay man" and its refutation have important social and legal implications. In 1996 I served on a jury in southern California trying a gay-bashing case. The defendant was accused of assaulting a young gay man in a bar. The defendant's lawyer tried to convince the jury that this gay man had made an unwanted pass at the defendant and thus "caused" the defendant to lose his temper and hit the gay man. I was surprised, but pleased and heartened that a jury of stolid working-class and middle-class citizens of varying ethnicities and ages did not find this argument convincing, and we convicted the defendant.[6] My experience gave me some hope that the power of this particular "excuse" for gay bashing is diminishing. *QE* does the same. It gives me hope that perhaps condoms—currently our best means of preventing life-threatening sexually transmitted diseases—will eventually make frequent but noneventful appearances on both cable and network TV shows and that they will be depicted as a simple fact of life for both gay and straight couples, as necessary and routine a part of life as the exfoliating scrub and moisturizer advocated by Kyan Douglas. I for one envision a day when the Fab Five will dispense, along with plasma televisions, leather furniture, theater tickets, and obscenely priced clothing, wisdom on reservoir tips and lubricant, and will provide all their straight guys with top-of-the-line condoms.

Moreover, *QE* is a hopeful sign that homophobia—the irrational hatred of homosexuality—and its attendant violence are losing ground in mainstream America. I would never argue that a television show could replace the hard work that must be done on the local and national level to ensure equality, civil rights, and personal safety for gays and lesbians. And I don't doubt that the popularity of the show hinges on gay men adhering to the social roles assigned them in popular culture; for example, hairdresser and interior decorator. But we must never, ever underestimate the power of our popular culture. As Michael Kimmel, a sociologist who studies masculinity and gender roles, notes: "It's a show premised on the collapse of homophobia among straight men. And in that sense *Queer Eye* may be doing more for gay rights than *Baker v. State* or *Lawrence v. Texas* ever could."[7] Does *QE* reinforce stereotypes? Possibly. Does it change some minds? That's a possibility as well. Does it depict straight men and gay men in friendly, flirty, cheerful social interaction—and could this qualify as a gay-straight dialogue? Absolutely! I am convinced that any TV show in which a straight guy's condoms and his "stick" are the subjects of gay humor is a show we should all be watching.

Acknowledgments

I would like to thank Karen Anijar and Thuy DaoJensen for their encouragement, their insightful comments on the first draft of this essay, and their capable editorship of this volume. I would also like to thank the students in my spring 2004 course "History of Sexuality in the United States" at Denison University. Their lively discussion about the social and cultural impact of *Queer Eye for the Straight Guy* helped inspire this essay.

Notes

[1] See Mark Simpson, "Here Come the Mirror Men," *The Independent*, November 12, 1994; and Mark Simpson, *Male Impersonators: Men Performing Masculinity* (London: Cassell Academic, 1997).

[2] Other readings are possible here. In her essay "We're So Sorry Uncle Gay Queer Alex" (forthcoming in M. Dalton and L. Linder, [Eds.], *The Sitcom Reader: America Viewed and Skewed*, Karen Anijar points out that gay men are almost always depicted in popular culture as

[3] And we must also acknowledge the implied threat to heterosexual authority. Cable television's Comedy Central recently debuted a reality TV show entitled *Straight Plan for the Gay Man*, a tongue-in-cheek attempt to reaffirm the cultural authority of straight men. Thanks to Karen Anijar to bringing this show to my attention.

[4] Andrea Tone, "Salute to Prophylaxis," in *Devices and Desires: A History of Contraceptives in America* (New York: Hill and Wang, 2001), pp. 91–115. For video clip from a military instruction film that encouraged sailors to use condoms during shore leave, see *Coming Out Under Fire* (1994).

[5] Bruce Steele, "The Gay Rights Makeover: How *Queer Eye for the Straight Guy*, armed with just paring knives and eyebrow pluckers, wins hearts and minds in the cause of equality," *The Advocate*, September 2, 2003, 42.

[6] In a much more widely publicized 1999 case, Aaron McKinney attempted to rationalize the savage beating that killed Mathew Shepard in Laramie, Wyoming, by claiming that he lost control when Shepard made a pass at him. The jury rejected that "defense" and convicted McKinney of murder.

[7] Michael Kimmel, "Gay-Straight Bonding on TV's *Queer Eye for the Straight Guy*," *Voice Male*, October 2003, 14.

Bibliography

Anijar, K. (2005, Forthcoming). We're so sorry uncle gay queer Alex. In M. Dalton and L. Linder, (Eds.), *The sitcom reader: America viewed and skewed.* Albany: State University of New York Press.

Kimmel, M. (2003). Gay-straight bonding on TV's *Queer Eye for the Straight Guy.*" *Voice Male*, October Issue: 14.

Simpson, M. (1994). Here Come the Mirror Men. *The Independent,* 12 November.

Simpson, M. (1997). *Male impersonators: Men performing masculinity.* London: Cassell Academic.

Tone, A. (2001). *Devices and desires: A history of contraceptives in America.* New York: Hill and Wang.

• CHAPTER FOUR •

Making Condoms Transgressive: *South Park* and "Proper Condom Use"

Mary M. Dalton

Amid the competing discourses on condom use in contemporary culture, none has gone so far as the animated hit comedy *South Park* to conflate the various arguments and effectively critique public discourse. Episode 507, "Proper Condom Use," manages to make condoms transgressive artifacts in a way that would seem unlikely, if not impossible, in a world that seems too "anything goes" to rightists and inhospitable to an open exchange of ideas and information to leftists. For some people, of course, condoms are inherently transgressive (see Anijar's chapter), but the pervasiveness of billboards and pamphlets and PSAs promoting safer sex practices has made prophylactics more public now than ever before (see Charlesworth's chapter). If we accept middle ground as a starting place for analyzing the strands of discourse surrounding condom use—not suggesting that there is anything approaching an actual consensus on the matter—then it is instructive to look at how this episode frames the debate. Essentially, "Proper Condom Use" employs excessive measures common to the serial narratives and necessary for this "transgressive" situation comedy to portray condoms as transgressive cultural artifacts, but at the same time different characters and groups of characters articulate various stands of discourse on sex education, from the serious to the nonsensical.

First, some background on the animated series. *South Park* has always been cast out of the mainstream, despite its popularity, because of its home network, rating, and time slot. *South Park* debuted on Comedy Central during the summer of 1997 with a TV-MA program rating, which designates it unsuitable for children under seventeen. The ten p.m. time slot and niche cable network home did not, however, stop the program from finding a dedicated audience; spawning a host of ancillary products featuring the one-dimensional, cutout figures of the main characters; and turning the four little boys into pop culture icons. The series centers on four nine-year-old boys living in a small Colorado mountain town. Stan, Kyle, Cartman, and Kenny are potty-mouthed boys who constantly raise issues that make the adult characters of the series uncomfortable. While the program is thought-provoking and decidedly clever in the way it contextualizes certain issues, the desire of the series creators to shock rather than enlighten creates a sort of virtual playground in which ideas are introduced but never fully interrogated; certainly none are championed.

Michael V. Tueth argues that transgressive humor, which is how he categorizes *South Park*, revels in folly rather than trying to dismantle it. Tueth writes:

> Unlike the intellectual wit and verbal sophistication of the satirical tradition, transgressive humor regresses to the infantile. Rather than portraying the objects of its humor in hopes that witty ridicule and public shame might provoke change, transgressive humor does not expect or even desire a change, for then the fun would end.
>
> Transgressive humor does share one element with satire. Both comic methods depend upon a basic consensus of standards and boundaries; otherwise, the joke would not be pleasurable. The societal taboos must remain, so that one can experience the delight of the entry into forbidden realms, a childish joy in simply breaking all the adult taboos, a pleasure indulged in for the sake of exposure of the impulses we have all been forced to repress.

That's not to say that transgressive humor doesn't sometimes serve some of the same purposes as satire by exposing and criticizing human ignorance, but actually effecting social change would cast *South Park* into another realm and eliminate its transgressive status.

The episode begins with little boys destroying a toy car carrying an image of an actual pop culture icon, Jennifer Lopez. As Kyle mouths lines ostensibly from the diva, "No, no, please! This time I *swear* I won't make albums or movies," Stan pulls a magnifying glass from his back pocket and fixes the sun's rays on the doll, which begins to melt and shrivel. Cartman runs up at this point to tell the others about how some older kids have taught him how to milk the dog, a game he calls "red rocket." While the others protest that dogs don't make milk, Cartman sexually stimulates the dog until it produces semen. This is significant because Stan interrupts his parents' book club meeting at home that night by replicating with Sparky, his family dog, what he had seen Cartman do earlier. The adults trying to discuss Steinbeck's *Cannery Row* are horrified, and Stan is sent to his room right away.

The "red rocket" game precipitates an embarrassed talk about sex at the Marsh household that night, a talk that will lead to the involvement of the *South Park* community. As this scene so aptly reveals, many parents are uncomfortable talking with their children about sexual topics and are eager to abdicate that task to institutions and organizations they feel are better equipped to handle these discussions.

>[Stan's house, later. His parents have entered his room, quite upset at his earlier behavior. Stan rests his head on his hands.]
>***Sharon:*** *Stanley, do you know why you're being grounded for ten months?*
>***Stan:*** *No!*
>***Randy:*** *Beating off the dog is not appropriate when we have company!* [Sharon glances at him.] *Ah I mean, ever! Beating off the dog is not appropriate ever!*
>***Stan:*** *Why?! What's the big deal?!*
>***Sharon:*** *Stanley, don't you understand what you are doing??*
>***Stan:*** *I was doing "red rocket" to make the dog's milk come out.*
>***Randy:*** *No, Stan! What you were doing to the dog was s-s-sexual.*
>***Stan:*** *Huh??*
>***Sharon:*** *You were stimulating the dog, Stanley! What came out of him was his...R-Randy?!*
>***Randy:*** *Well, you know, when you do that to a m-male...the...eh, eh...you make his...stuff come out.* [Stan looks confused.] *Well, Jesus, haven't they taught you these things at school?*
>***Stan:*** *What things??*
>***Sharon:*** *Sexual education. Haven't you learned that yet?*
>***Stan:*** *No!*
>***Sharon:*** *Oh. Look, well, you see, Stanley...Well, your school should be teaching this stuff!*
>***Randy:*** *Yeah! Let's get that damned school on the phone!*
>[Randy walks out the door. Sharon follows him out. Stan looks ahead blankly.]

Later, at the *South Park* PTA meeting, it becomes clear that Sharon and Randy Marsh are not alone. Rather than accept responsibility for giving their children information at home appropriate for their maturity level and consistent with their family's values, most parents seem to agree with Sharon when she stands up and says, "Look, our kids are learning sexual things on the street and on television. There's no way we can stop it. The schools have to teach them sexual education at a younger age." School administrators, represented by Principal Victoria, seem to want to balance the interests of the group with the stated policy that sexual education begins in the fifth grade, and, despite cautionary warnings from Chef, those in charge heed the parents' demands and implement an expansion of the sexual education curriculum to include even the youngest children at the school. It is in this way that the episode represents the voices of parents who want to cede the responsibility for teaching their children about sex because they are uncomfortable talking about it but realize the importance of the subject—they do not want to talk to their own children but, paradoxically, understand that someone must talk with them.

Each of the strands of discourse in the episode related to sex education—and, by extension, to condoms—contains a similar paradox, which adds another layer of complexity to the narrative. Following this pattern, "Proper Condom Use" also represents the discourse of school administrators who are swayed by public opinion (in this case in favor of broadening sex education) in the heat of a controversy. The administrators try to figure out how to appease parents to avoid controversy, but end up, as we shall see, offering instruction that thoroughly confuses the children and causes the major controversy they had hoped to avoid.

This technique of introducing a thread of discourse amid competing threads, then disrupting *each* thread to effect a paradox, is exploited most effectively with the three teacher characters who are charged with teaching sex education: Ms. Choksondik (pronounced chokes-ON-dick) teaches "abstinence only" to fourth-grade girls; Mr. Mackey tries to teach the basics of biological principles and responsible sex practices to fourth-grade boys; and Mr. Garrison espouses an intentionally explicit and age-inappropriate discourse with a kindergarten class.

Ms. Choksondik uses scare tactics focusing on sexually transmitted diseases (STDs) and pregnancy to drive the girls into a panic.

> ***Ms. Choksondik:*** *All right, girls, even though this may be stuff you don't want to hear, you need to hear it.*
> ***Wendy:*** *Oh, we* wanna *hear it, Ms. Choksondik. We're excited.*
> ***Bebe:*** *Yeah, we think it's gonna be fun!*
> ***Girls:*** *Yeah!*
> ***Ms. Choksondik:*** *Fun! It's going to be fun! Well, let's start with our first lesson, then, shall we?* [writes on the board] *SEXUALLY TRANSMITTED DISEASES!* [The girls sit quietly.] *That's right, because unless you get boys to wear condoms you can and will get a sexually transmitted disease from them! How fun is that, hmmm?! Is that fun?*

Wendy: I didn't mean that—
Ms. Choksondik: Today over twenty thousand Americans will contract a sexual disease! TODAY! Twelve thousand more tomorrow! And the reason is that you girls wake up in the morning and say, "It's not going to happen to me." You say, "Oh, Ms. Choksondik, that happens to girls in Detroit, in Brooklyn, but not here in Colorado." WRONG! [The girls look chastened.] *Gonorrhea, herpes, chlamydia, HPV, HIV, syphilis, hepatitis B, hepatitis C, the list goes on and on! These are serious diseases! They have serious consequences!* [The girls are definitely afraid.] *You think that sex is about fun and games and love?* [now with a folder in her left hand] *Wrong! Sex is about disease! Here's a little picture of herpes.*
Girls: AAAHHH!
Ms. Choksondik: And here's a little syphilis for you!
Girls: AAAHHH!
Ms. Choksondik: That's right, girls. Here's what happens when you don't get boys to use condoms!

The girls then run in terror from their male classmates in the cafeteria and the playground, telling them not to come closer unless they are wearing their condoms and launching what will turn out to be a literal battle between the fourth-grade sexes.

At first the boys are baffled. After all, their first sex education class was with the hapless Mr. Mackey. He began the class period by saying anatomically correct words for male and female sex organs amid boyish giggles, then stumbling at the point of describing actual intercourse. When Stan asks the nervous teacher whether he's actually had intercourse, Mr. Mackey replies, "Well, sure I have! It's just…I was about nineteen at the time, so it's been about twenty-one years…." When the girls do ask later about the condoms, the boys realize that, as Stan puts it, "Dude, Mr. Mackey didn't know anything about anything," and they decide to go to the South Park Pharmacy to buy condoms.

The pharmacist (male) and assistant (female) represent a discourse of health education, but they contradict one another and present another paradox as ten fourth-grade boys line up at the counter to buy condoms. The pharmacist asks their age, with evident concern, and is surprised by the answer.

Pharmacist: Sorry, kids, I'm not selling you condoms.

Kyle: Well, why not? You want us to get AIDS?
Pharmacist: I just don't think kids your age should be—
Assistant: [intervening] Mark, we have to be willing to supply condoms to anyone who requests them.
Mark: But...they're...children!
Assistant: Would you rather them do it unprotected?
Cartman: Yeah, you want us unprotected, asshole?
Mark: I just think that all this sex ed and condom talk in elementary school is wrong!
Assistant: Kids are going to do what they do, and it's up to us to make sure they're protected.
Stan: Well, I'm glad this lady's on our side.
Mark: I don't think we have any that'll even fit them!
Assistant: Sure we do. We just got in the new Gladiators for kids. Li'l Minis. They're specially designed for kids under ten, and they're only five ninety-five for a box of fifty.
Butters: Fifty? Uh, can't we just use the same one every day?
Assistant: No, you have to change it.
Kyle: Oh, jeez, we're gonna have to buy tons of these things.

Both the pharmacist and the assistant appear comfortable with the clinical aspects of their jobs. The pharmacist, however, tries to temper his comments with reason, while the chirpy assistant (as she is identified in the script, although there is no visual cue that she is not a second pharmacist) is ready to follow the stated policy, even though giving condoms to nine-year-olds seems absurd. But is it absurd in the universe of *South Park*? Apparently not, since there is a new product manufactured specifically for "kids under ten." This is more than a plot device that facilitates the purchase of condoms by the children and, eventually, the all-out war that will be waged between the boys and the girls; Li'l Minis at $5.95 for a box of fifty serve to make the condom itself a transgressive artifact for the audience viewing the situation comedy. What would it take in our own culture, where condoms have become ubiquitous, to make them shocking? Something like producing and marketing prophylactics for elementary school children would serve that end. The pharmacist, however well-meaning, and the assistant, however efficient and chirpy, are like the other adults in the episode: They are talking *to* one another and talking *at* the children—but they are not listening to the children.

Ms. Choksondik and Mr. Mackey have been stimulated by all the sex talk to a growing awareness of one another and decide to get together to discuss lesson plans for upcoming classes. Two conventionally unattractive cut-out figure teachers—who remind us in stature of Jack Spratt and his wife—come together in what is surely the most ironic sequence of the episode. Sparked by the sex talk and encouraged by respective revelations about their lack of popularity in high school and after (Ms. Choksondik has never had sex), the two end up making out. Soon their clothes come off and foreplay begins in earnest. At the critical moment just before intercourse, Ms. Choksondik has the presence of mind to ask Mr. Mackey if he has a condom, and he replies "Well. No." When their cartoon eyes meet, the teacher who earlier had admonished the girls about the terrible things that would happen to them if the boys didn't wear condoms gives in to her passion with a decisive, "Oh well, fuck it." His was the voice of responsible behavior and hers the voice of abstinence, but their actions as they engage in "unprotected" sex with great gusto form the paradox that disrupts both threads of discourse.

Meanwhile, the boys are wearing their condoms so the girls will talk to them, and reports from the South Park Pharmacy about rampant sexual activity among fourth graders (assumptions based on condom purchases) cause school administrators to authorize sex education for younger students. When Principal Victoria inquires, "But how old do you think a student should be when they learn about proper condom use?" Ms. Choksondik has a ready reply: kindergarten. In the next scene, Mr. Garrison demonstrates putting a Gladiator condom on a model phallus with his mouth, which astonishes the children around the table and finally causes one of the boys to cry. Mr. Garrison is later identified by Chef as a "complete pervert," and his presence in the episode seems designed expressly to push the boundaries and extend the threads of discourse represented to include something so far outside the mainstream and beyond the margins of society that it is, along with the Li'l Minis, a transgressive discourse. Mr. Garrison's message to the tiny tots seems to be that anything goes, but he really is suggesting by topics discussed that sex education only includes the mechanics of "kinky" acts, all of which are clearly inappropriate for children of any age. Certainly, his presence in the classroom and the topics he discusses are included solely for shock value and are not to be taken seriously.

When the boys discover that they have been unwittingly duped by the girls into wearing condoms unnecessarily, they are furious. In class one day, Mr. Mackey learns that the boys are wearing the condoms around the clock.

Mr. Mackey: *Why are you wearing a condom?*
Cartman: *So I don't get AIDS.*

> *Mr. Mackey: Eric, you can't get AIDS from just sitting around, you have to get it from sex.*
> *Stan: From sex?*
> *Mr. Mackey: Yes.*
> *Kyle: You mean, intercourse with a girl?*
> *Mr. Mackey: Yes! Now will you all pay attention, please? The vagina and the clitoris are on the outside, and they are in fact very easily visible to the naked eye.*
> *Stan: All this time...It's the girls that give us diseases!*
> *Cartman: I knew it! Girls lie! They lie right to your face!*
> *Mr. Mackey: Now here we can see the interior female anatomy. Things like the uterus and the ovaries are on the inside*
> *Kyle: Well, that does it! If us boys are going to live, we have to get rid of the girls!*
> *Stan: Yeah, come on guys, this is war!* [leaves his seat and heads for the door. The other boys follow.]
> *Boys:* [among their statements] *Yeah! That's right! Come on!*

The boys gather and attack a stronghold that the girls have built to keep them at bay. It is all-out war, with a girl firing a Gatling gun, boys hurling a Molotov cocktail, and other weapons used rampantly. Finally, a much larger explosion rouses the adults of *South Park* and draws them to the wreckage.

Amid some finger-pointing comes a sheepish admission from Ms. Choksondik: "I'm afraid this is all my fault. I...think I went a little overboard scaring the girls. I forgot to tell them that to get diseases from boys you...have to have sex with them first." The kids finally "get it" and utter a collective "Oooohhh." Just as the light dawns on the children that the information they received lacked the proper context for them to understand what it all meant, Chef takes center stage to give the "meaningful speech" of the episode before undercutting his own dialogue. Notably, Chef is the only person of color in the town, and it is also notable that the only African-American character in the town is voiced by the baritone soul singer Isaac Hayes. The casting of Hayes, who won an Academy Award for Best Original Song for a Motion Picture in 1970 for "Theme from *Shaft*," seems an intentional exploitation of the negative stereotype of the oversexed black. In episode after episode, Chef is constantly discussing sex with the little boys of *South Park* and often says a little too much before realizing that the boys do not fully understand what he is telling them. There is an illustrative example in "Proper Condom Use":

• Making Condoms Transgressive •   45

> [The school kitchen, lunch.]
> ***Chef:*** *Hello there, children.*
> ***Boys:*** *Hey, Chef.*
> ***Chef:*** *How is sexual education class going?*
> ***Stan:*** *It's dumb. Mr. Mackey doesn't teach us nothin'.*
> ***Chef:*** *Yeah, I don't think Ol' Mackey knows a hymen from a hysterectomy. And Choksondik? I'd be surprised if she's ever gotten laid in her life.*
> ***Kyle:*** *Yeah...Chef, what's "laid"?*
> ***Chef:*** *Oh, nothin'. Now, move along, children, you're holdin' up the line.*

Even so, the school cafeteria worker is the rare adult in *South Park* who listens to the boys and seems to have their best interests at heart.

Throughout "Proper Condom Use," Chef provides a voice of reason drowned out by the near-hysteria of parents who do not want to accept the responsibility for talking to their children about sex. He speaks twice during the PTA meeting near the beginning of the episode.

> ***Principal Victoria:*** *School policy has been to teach sexual education later. In the fifth grade.*
> ***Mr. Tweek:*** *It isn't soon enough.*
> ***Stuart:*** *Yeah. Why, just this afternoon our son was caught beatin' off our dog.*
> [Randy and Sharon look at each other in recognition of the act.]
> ***Chef:*** *Look, parents. Do you really want your children learning about sex? Part of the fun of being a kid is being naive! Let them be kids for a while.*
> ***Ms. Choksondik:*** *Naive at what cost, Chef? Parents, we have to face facts: Children in America are having sex at younger and younger ages. STDs are affecting younger and younger kids all the time. The only way we can combat that is by educating children before they have sex.*
> ***Chef:*** *The first thing that kids learn about sex shouldn't be some bitch-scare tactic about STDs.*
> ***Sheila:*** [rising] *No, she's right! With all the teen pregnancies that are out today, I think my boy* does *need to know about sexual education.* [sits, then rises again] *From the school.*
> ***Adults:*** *Yeah. Uh-huh. Yeah, we have to.*

While the parents are unwilling to listen to Chef during the South Park PTA meeting, they are shocked into silence long enough to consider his words after the massive gender war at the stronghold, which is now a burning wreckage.

> ***Chef:*** *Well, I hate to say it, but you all got what you deserved.*
> ***Parents:*** *Huh?*
> ***Chef:*** *Look. Schools are teaching condom use to younger and younger students each day! But sex isn't something that should be taught in textbooks and diagrams. Sex is emotional and spiritual. It needs to be taught by family. I know it can be hard, parents, but if you leave it up to the schools to teach sex to kids, you don't know who they're learning it from. It could be from someone who doesn't know* [a shot of Mr. Mackey], *someone who has a bad opinion of it* [a shot of Ms. Choksondik looking around], *or even a complete pervert* [a shot of Mr. Garrison].

Of course, now that Chef has finally been established as the voice of reason, it is time for him to follow in the wake of the other characters, all of whom disrupt their respective threads of discourse with some paradoxical action or statement. When Stan asks his friend when is the right age for him and his friends to start having sex, Chef offers a simplistic answer that belies the wisdom of his earlier statements.

> ***Chef:*** *It's very simple, children. The right time to start having sex is* [close-up] *seventeen.*
> ***Kyle:*** *Seventeen?*
> [Sheila and Gerald approach.]
> ***Chef:*** *Seventeen.*
> ***Sheila:*** *So you mean seventeen as long as you're in love?*
> ***Chef:*** *Nope, just seventeen.*
> ***Gerald:*** *But what if you're not ready at seventeen?*
> ***Chef:*** *Seventeen! You're ready.*

With this statement punctuating Chef's previous statements advocating prudence and responsibility, once again a contradiction in the text erases attempts by the viewer to attribute some larger meaning to the narrative that might point toward a unified ideology on the part of the creators or suggest some prescriptive for the larger culture with regard to sex education.

The idea that there is no single message in "Proper Condom Use" beyond shocking the audience and calling into question all threads of discourse on sex education for children is reinforced in the narrative by the children characters themselves. The children at South Park Elementary School have no particular agenda; they do not represent any of the threads of discourse on sex education either individually or in groups. Interestingly, the children seem neither negatively nor positively influenced by the inability of their parents to assume responsibility for talking with them about sex and by the ineptitude of the various school personnel at implementing a curriculum to give them the accurate and balanced information they might need. Before the embers have cooled at the devastated stronghold, Cartman announces, "Well, I guess now that that's out of the way, we can get on with our lives," and he approaches a dog that has entered the scene to play "red rocket." The point of this series is, perhaps, consciously anti-didactic just as it is clearly transgressive. In this episode, condoms are the artifact of choice for pushing boundaries and for *almost* making points about the larger culture. While critics can critique the careful artlessness of *South Park*'s visual style, the intentional vulgarity of the scripts, and the dearth of easy answers about how to solve compelling social problems, most would agree that the series raises revealing and relevant questions central to our process of understanding ourselves and our culture.

Bibliography

South Park (2001). Transcript from Episode #507. Available from: *www.southpark.dsl.pipex.com/scripts/scr507.shtml*

Tueth, M. V. (2005, Forthcoming). Breaking and entering: Transgressive comedy on television. In M. Dalton and L. Linder (Eds.), *The sitcom reader: America viewed and skewed.* Albany: State University of New York Press.

• CHAPTER FIVE •

Don't Avoid or Make Void the Topic

Chris Bell

It sounds so simple. Wear a condom and you just might save your life. Of course there are select circumstances where this maxim does not apply, for instance if the condom has a design imperfection (read: a hole or tear) and/or if it is improperly used. Nonetheless, there is something appealing in the notion that a simple rubber device extends longevity.

This essay chronicles my experience with that life-saving rubber device, the condom: from one of the first times I touched one to the occasions I wish I had used one. I describe the mistakes I made, but only with the understanding that, in the final analysis, I choose not to harbor any regrets. If anything, I feel fortunate to reflect on these episodes and commit them to paper in the hopes that the reader will think about my experiences and perhaps learn from my mistakes.

Ten Years Ago
I have been assigned the task of preparing and delivering a ten-minute informative speech for my Public Speaking class. It's odd—most of my classmates are upperclassmen who have postponed this required course for as long as possible. I, on the other hand, enrolled in Public Speaking as a freshman because I thought it would be fun, standing in front of an audience, discussing timely and intriguing topics. Although this is college, where the scholarly expectations are high, I see nothing wrong with infusing a little humor into the proceedings.

With this in mind, I spend several days brainstorming ideas. What topic of interest might I select that will maintain the requisite level of academic exactitude, yet include a tangible tinge of humor? The widespread popularity and appeal of Fox's often-crass but undeniably funny variety show *In Living Color*? The cultural significance of TLC, the new R&B trio whose members affix condoms to their clothes? I consider a wealth of topics, dismissing all of them as too esoteric, mundane, or complex to develop substantively in a ten-minute speech.

One night, while listening to a Top Ten countdown show on the radio, the DJ's stentorian voice booms forth: "Tonight's number seven song is a re-entry from a few months ago. I dunno why you guys out there in Listener Land are requesting this one, but here it is." The tune in question is Salt-N-Pepa's *Let's Talk About Sex*. Remembering this song as *the* jam from the previous semester, I begin to get into the groove:

Let's talk about sex right now to the people at home or in the crowd
It keeps coming up anyhow
Don't decoy, avoid or make void the topic
Cuz that ain't gonna stop it

After the song concludes, and the DJ gleefully introduces Right Said Fred's *I'm Too Sexy*, I consider Salt-N-Pepa's musical treatise. A rap ditty that unabashedly urges listeners to have serious conversations with their partners about sex, the song is neither preachy nor overly didactic. One line in the song emphasizes the importance of condom usage. Taking that lyric as my cue, I spontaneously decide to devote my informative speech to the topic of how to use a condom.

The next morning, I proceed to the university's library to plot my course of action. I figure I should include some information about the consequences of incorrectly using a condom or just not using one at all; thus, I begin by researching STD and AIDS statistics. In the process, I come across the toll-free number of the Centers for Disease Control. That evening, I speak to a CDC information specialist, gleaning additional statistics and locations of STD and HIV testing venues in my community. After our conversation ends, I create a handout of this information in the residence hall computer lab.

During the next few days, I design and practice my speech. I start by discussing how college students are engaging in sexual activity more often than many of us care to consider. Next, I outline AIDS trends as well as the prevalence of sexually transmitted diseases in college and university communities. I conclude by demonstrating how to protect oneself by using a condom. The day before I am scheduled to deliver my speech, I go to the Student Health Center to acquire a box of free condoms. I marvel at the ease with which I flash my student ID and procure the prophylactics, saving me a budget-busting $3.99. That night I sit on my dorm room floor with my Public Speaking textbook, index cards, handouts, and the condoms strewn around me. Midway through my final practice run, my roommate, Perry, enters the room. The sight of me sitting there alone with an exposed condom in one hand and a bottle of K-Y jelly in the other clearly, *hopefully*, strikes him as unusual.

Don't Avoid or Make Void the Topic

To his credit, Perry does not betray his curiosity, opting instead to step over me with nothing more than a "Hey...um...how was your day?"

As luck would have it, I am selected to present first on the pivotal day. Standing in front of the class in my suit and tie (this is for a grade!), I scarcely need to refer to my carefully inscribed index cards. I have rehearsed the introductory material and statistics so thoroughly during the preceding week that the information has embedded itself in my memory as firmly as my own name. Then comes the fun part.

"Now I've just described how STDs and AIDS are affecting college-age populations. At this point, I'm going to move into the heart of my speech by showing you how to protect yourselves by properly placing a condom on the penis. For this part of my presentation, I need a volunteer, preferably male."

There is utter silence. The student who had been well on her way to Dreamland sits up with a jolt, eyes snapping wide open. My professor raises an eyebrow. No one volunteers. Consternation uninhibitedly colors my face.

"C'mon, you guys, I'm getting graded here. Can somebody help me out?"

Nervous giggles penetrate the audience's silence.

Sighing in frustration, I remark, "Well, Mama said I should always be prepared to rely on myself. Here goes nothing."

I calmly stroll around the table, positioning myself behind the podium where I had strategically hidden a banana before anyone in the class arrived. The banana is at crotch level. Accordingly, it appears I am toying with my own anatomy while readying the piece of fruit. To prolong the suspense, I mumble, "I'll just need a second here to get things, um, ready."

"Oh my God," one of my classmates drawls. "I can't believe him," another declares.

"Okay, here we go. This is the male penis..."

I shove aside the podium with a deliriously over-the-top flourish. Several female coeds scream and pretend to cover their eyes. My professor stands in protest. When they realize I am merely holding a banana, everyone collapses into uproarious, unabated laughter. Their mirth is certainly justified, considering this particular banana is so robust one would presume it has been injected with anabolic steroids. Additionally, the banana features the most unusual curve in its composition. I had spent some quality time in the Wal-Mart produce section the previous afternoon looking for the perfect specimen.

"...and this is the condom." Reaching into my pocket, I extract an unwrapped condom. I begin my demonstration, during which my peers continually express amusement and guffaws at my enormous "penis." "Gently tear open the condom wrapper, never with your teeth, no matter how, er, hungry you are. Check for tears and apply the lubricant of choice, but not Vaseline—or Valvoline, for that matter. Next, unroll the condom completely and place it around the length of the penis."

I accomplish this latter part, but not without pronounced difficulty. I haven't actually practiced this chief component of my presentation as much as I should have or as much as I have rehearsed the other parts. Indeed, I never bothered to read the instructions clearly printed on the box of condoms—the instructions that indicate how to place a condom on a penis correctly, by unrolling it down the length of the shaft while simultaneously holding the condom's tip and squeezing out air bubbles. As a result, I stand in front of my classmates and professor and demonstrate how NOT to use a condom, obliviously maneuvering my banana-penis into the unrolled prophylactic.

Despite this grave error, I receive a hearty round of applause from my classmates upon conclusion. (Looking back, I realize they were most likely feting my *chutzpah* and the humor I had integrated, not my dexterity or the [lack of] efficacy with which I demonstrated how to use a condom.) Not surprisingly, any bad feelings I might have sensed about my improper demonstration are swiftly discounted when, at the conclusion of the class period, I receive my grade on the speech: an A-plus.

*   *   *   *   *

A few hours later, I sit in my dorm room studying for a history examination while the Top Ten countdown airs in the background. It has been a little over a week since I heard *Let's Talk About Sex*, the song that inspired my speech. The tune is not played on the request-based countdown that evening. It has fallen off. In retrospect, I wonder if the sentiment had as well.

Eight Years Ago
It is Spring Break during my junior year. Having completely come to terms with my (homo)sexuality in the midst of a tumultuous sophomore year, I am now seeking camaraderie—another gay man to talk to, to spend time with, to date. This is what is foremost on my mind as I drive to Forest Park in St. Louis.

I began frequenting Forest Park the previous summer, after a friend advised me that this was a place where gay men hung out. My definition of "hanging out" ultimately proved different from that of the other assembled gentlemen. I expected to see guys talking with each other about music, movies, and the like. Perhaps two men would exchange phone numbers and meet for a dinner date. I soon realized how naive my expectations were, as this was, above all else, a place where men came to fuck. This realization turned me off, until I learned to console myself in the belief that since I visited the park in the hopes of meeting someone for a platonic relationship, surely there must be one other individual looking for the same thing. It was with this thought firmly in mind that I made return appearances to Forest Park whenever I was home on break.

On this occasion, I am sitting in my car listening to Janet Jackson's *If* on the radio. Although the song is a year old, it still maintains its infectiousness. I'm embarrassed to cherish the song given its sexually explicit nature, but I do. Midway through Janet's opus, I notice I am being cruised by a guy in a red Pontiac. He glances over at me. When I return his gaze, he swiftly looks away. When I drive off, he follows me, hovering nearby after I've settled elsewhere for a continuation of the "eye game." This activity repeats itself for several long, tense minutes. Eventually, we pull up side by side.

"So, are you in the mood for a little sixty-nine?"

His bluntness takes me aback. Not to mention that this is not the sort of conversation or activity I am looking for. So I smile, firmly shake my head to decline, put the car in gear, and am on my way.

I drive home and eat dinner. While picking over my food, I think to myself, "Tomorrow I'll be twenty years old. If I can't be in a dating relationship with a man, at least I can say I've had a sexual relationship with one." I also realize I can either give this a try or spend the remainder of my break watching *Ricki Lake*. Immediately I place my plate in the kitchen sink, grab my car keys, and make it to Forest Park in record time.

Mr. Red Pontiac is still there. After I pull up next to him, I say, "I changed my mind."

"I was just about to leave," he replies. "Why don't I meet you here tomorrow at eleven a.m.?"

"Fine."

I want camaraderie, but I am willing to settle.

*　　*　　*　　*　　*

We meet at the park the next day. I follow him to his home in the Central West End, one of the ostensibly "gayer" neighborhoods in St. Louis. He lives in a beautiful condo, well-apportioned and superbly decorated. When I comment on the latter, he smiles and says, "I should hope so. I'm a decorator."

He does not strike me as anxious or ill at ease. Conversely, I am a nervous wreck. While he gives me the grand tour, my thoughts are on the Forest Park sting operation I had read about some time before wherein the police entrapped gay men in park bathrooms, arresting them for indecent exposure and public lewdness. I figure he can't be an undercover cop because we've come too far. Instead, I choose to brand him as a murderer, which doesn't do much to heighten my sense of security.

The tour concludes in the master bedroom. He sits on the bed while I linger in the doorway. After we engage in the smallest talk possible, he pats the bed beside him. As I walk over to be with him, my thoughts are on him killing me with a gun, a knife, or some other tangible weapon of choice. It does not occur to me that he can just as easily kill me with a virus.

Seconds later, I push all thoughts of mortality from my mind. In their place, I revel in the knowledge that he is eighteen years older than I am, he is beautiful, and he wants me. Me! He puts a condom on. Everything—and I do mean everything—seems fine.

* * * * *

Driving past Forest Park later that afternoon, I realize I will not be returning. There is nothing else there for me. As I head home, I begin singing, "Happy birthday to me."

Seven Years Ago
It is one month before I graduate from college. Among other concerns, the memory of my Forest Park tryst weighs heavily on my mind. One evening while watching Greg Louganis discuss his HIV-positive status on *20/20*, I am galvanized to seek testing. Although Mr. Red Pontiac and I had used a pair of condoms, one for each go-round, I am still nervous.

The next month, I march across the stage and accept my degree, an HIV-negative person whose mind is at ease.

Six Years Ago
I am in the first year of graduate school. My classes are engaging, I've made a slew of new friends, and George Michael has an irresistibly danceable single out about casual sex called *Fast Love*. One night, I am in the local gay

bar dancing to that song when I notice a strikingly good-looking gentleman. When George's voice fades, I ask a friend to introduce us. His name is Todd.

Todd and I share an instant, animalistic attraction to one another. Within the hour, we reconnoiter at his house to have sex—taking every precaution you could think of. Hey, I'm no fool. I've already had one HIV scare. So after Todd expertly slips the condom on, it's all good.

Five Years Ago
I have reached the second and final year of my master's program. My life is unusually hectic: I have a stack of Freshman Composition papers to grade, thesis research to accomplish, Ph.D. applications to fill out, and a Canterbury Tale to read. Did I mention I need to finish these tasks this week? Before I can fully devote my attention to these concerns, I have an appointment at the Student Health Center to receive my test results. Two weeks ago, I ventured to Student Health because my lymph nodes remained swollen and engorged from a bout with mononucleosis one month earlier. The doctor informed me I should not be alarmed, perhaps some of the mono virus was still in my system. Just to be on the safe side, she suggested I have tests for lymphoma, Parkinson's disease, and HIV.

The doctor enters the examination room and manages a weak smile. She takes a seat next to me. "All of your tests are negative except one," she states. "The HIV antibody test came back positive."

While she moves into post-test counseling (phrases such as "T-cell count," "viral load," and "drug regimen" pepper her monologue), I no longer think about all the work I have to do. It strikes me as trivial now. I choose not to think about how Todd and I stopped using condoms midway through the year and a half we spent together because he falsely told me our relationship was a monogamous one. I do not think about what I am going to tell my mom. Instead, my thoughts are strangely but significantly occupied with all the pop culture warning signs I neglected: One of my favorite episodes of *Designing Women* when Suzanne Sugarbaker remarks that Tony Goldwyn's character, the interior decorator, contracted HIV because he did not "use protection"; Salt-N-Pepa remixing *Let's Talk About Sex* into *Let's Talk About AIDS* for a public service announcement; Janet Jackson coyly albeit pointedly prefacing her song *If* with an admonition to her partner to "Be a good boy and put this [condom] on"; TLC's groundbreaking *Waterfalls* video, which includes a compelling sequence about a hunky guy who dies from AIDS after having sex without a condom.

But I suppose all that is irrelevant at this moment. I should be listening to what the doctor is saying to me. Nonetheless, I can't help recalling these pop culture touchstones, these messages I wantonly (a)voided, wondering how I could be so naive as to think they were not intended for me.

Eventually, the doctor asks me how I am feeling. My thoughts turn to the pivotal scene in *Evita* when Colonel Peron informs his beloved she is dying. Her response underscores my feelings during those taut moments in the Student Health Center:

So what happens now/
Where am I going to?

Last Year
I am in Chicago, my home since leaving graduate school. For various reasons, I did not complete my master's degree. I have not enrolled in a Ph.D. program. I am not engaged with any of the activities I anticipated doing at this stage in my life. Instead, I travel the country speaking to high school and college students about HIV/AIDS.

Today, I am reading the *Chicago Tribune* on the subway as I head to O'Hare Airport. There is a small article relaying a recently released statistic from the Centers for Disease Control: 7 percent of white gay and bisexual men in the United States are HIV-positive compared with 33 percent of black gay and bisexual men. This epidemiological data has been culled from surveys in six urban centers and is indicative of a "new and alarming" trend in AIDS policy. I toss the paper aside in frustration.

I am frustrated because I used to call the CDC for AIDS statistics and now I am one. I am frustrated because I would rather have received a failing grade on my Public Speaking assignment if someone had simply pointed out my error in placing the condom on the banana. At least then I would have known. I am frustrated that in my junior year in college, I enrolled in a class on HIV/AIDS prevention and education and received a solid A. Nevertheless, I still engaged in unprotected sexual intercourse for a period of several months. I guess that's proof of the virtual chasm between theory and practice, that a person can be equipped with knowledge but there is no guarantee he will apply what he has learned. I am frustrated that the average lifespan of an HIV-positive person is ten years; thus, for all intents and purposes, I should be dead by my thirty-third birthday, five years from now. And I am frankly pissed about this CDC statistic warning of "a new trend" for black gay and bisexual men—as if *all of a sudden*, we're becoming infected at rapid rates. As a black, gay, HIV-positive person, it is clear to me there is a need for massive intervention, including education on properly using condoms.

I do not buy into the ideology that there is one tried-and-true method of promoting effective condom use. "Wear a rubber" might work for Liz, the suburban socialite, but there is nothing to suggest that same message will be equally efficacious for Mookie from the 'hood. This is why cultural indicators, e.g., music, safer sex ad campaigns, and celebrities revealing their HIV status have the potential to impact what people do in their most intimate moments. People respond differently to protection messages. There was a time when I could recite every lyric to *Let's Talk About Sex*, but I could not discern that Salt-N-Pepa were including me in their rap. To that end, there should be a wealth of ways to promote the urgency of condom use. There should also be strategies to measure the success of these endeavors as well as a willingness to address lapses in public policy. Why, for example, are so many gay men engaging in unprotected sex? Why has this population invented a "brave and daring" euphemism for this action, "barebacking"? How many more individuals must become infected with HIV and die from AIDS before the message that condoms are not a passing fancy but a priority in our climate is finally ingrained?

Yet despite all of the AIDS statistics, the disease's staggering death toll, and the proven efficacy of condoms, there are still elected officials, clergy, and others who are reticent to have discussions about condoms and/or make them widely available. People are dying, but the United States, with its immense wealth and power, has yet to devise a viable course of action. It seems to me that if the United States has the resources to bomb other nations on a whim, then there can be a resolution to the dilemma of this country's lack of an effective AIDS prevention policy.

* * * * *

When I am invited to a high school or university to speak about HIV/AIDS, I ask at the outset if I may distribute condoms. I explain that I am reluctant to speak at a venue that will not allow me to do so because it would be simultaneously disingenuous and hypocritical for me not to promote effective condom use. There has been only one instance in which the organizers at a host institution had a problem with this. As I proceeded to the stage, they adamantly stated that I could pass out red ribbons, but nothing more. The red ribbon, incredible symbol that it is, is just that—a symbol, an adornment. A condom, on the other hand, can be used. It is a life-saving tool.

This is what I said that afternoon as I began to pass out condoms and the organizers cast embittered, caustic glances in my direction.

Moreover, no matter where I speak, from Boise State in Idaho to the University of Delaware, I notice one similarity. Whenever I reach the point in my story about how Todd and I stopped using condoms, someone nods. People understand where I am coming from when I state that Todd and I never had a conversation about not using condoms. One night, we just didn't. Nor did we the next time we were together. Perhaps this is indicative of a typical way people stop using protection? Perhaps this action underscores a link between the emotional place of the relationship and condom use? Perhaps not using condoms is a symbol, valid or not, of monogamy? In any event, Todd and I continued to make the same mistake over and over again until it became a natural part of our sex practices. By the time we discussed it, by the time Todd came up with the monogamy lie, it seemed to make little difference. But what a difference it could have made.

* * * * *

I come out of my solemn reverie in time to hear the conductor state, "This is O'Hare, as far as this train goes. All passengers must exit the train." I grab my luggage and disembark. As I proceed down the platform toward the terminal, I begin practicing the stoic expression I will don in a few moments when the screener x-rays my carry-on bag and sees that it is filled to bursting with male and female condoms and lubricant.

Tomorrow
"Good evening. My name is Chris Bell. I was invited here to speak with you about HIV and AIDS, more specifically, my experiences living with HIV. I suppose the easiest way to delve into all of this would be to go back to about ten years ago when I was a freshman in college...."

• CHAPTER SIX •

Exchanging Fluid Discourses of Social Dis-ease: Visual Cultural Studies as Prophylactic Praxis as Rough Trade

James H. Sanders

The necessary tension between the longing embedded in people's desire for a fuller life, [and] a more complete self...is almost unspeakable. [W]hat cannot be contained is allowed to live through the form of art. This is why at times art is perceived as subversive...because it reminds people of what has been buried—desires their deepest selves dream but cannot manifest within the existing system. —Becker (1994, 118)

In the late twentieth century, too few artists and art educators have been rising to the challenge of addressing social dis-ease concerning sexual discourses. Aroused by students' unprotected sharing of fluid concepts regarding multiple indentificatory possibilities, this short paper fingers the risks involved in mounting concerns socially constructed as filthy, untouchable, and dangerous. Amidst crisis discourses (Singer, 1993) and the spread of epidemic logic concerning not only HIV-AIDS, but also arts-marginality in the curriculum, intellectual sluts like myself have entered the rough trade of exploring the power dynamics around sexuality, morality, ethics, art, and politics in education curriculum through performative gestures and intentionally provocative language texts. With screams of (dis)pleasure voiced by colleagues and (under)graduates as I roughback these issues through intellectually promiscuous readings and pedagogical practices—I momentarily pull myself out of that moist and heated space, smoke a cigarette, and take pleasure in reflecting on the dangers of exposing my unsheathed concepts to diseased minds too tight to accommodate the fullness of my political passion.

My experience of using the naked body in performance art to arouse thinking about the dangers of research that explores the researcher's intimate knowledge of the personal/political dynamics in the arts teaching/learning context is, for some, a pleasurable awakening of performative possibilities—and for others, a fluid and dangerous proposition that may be perceived as exhibitionism. At first I believed that transforming political performative gestures into printed word would serve as a prophylactic—containing the fluid concepts so streams of theoretical and narrative research could be felt without demanding they be swallowed. But in advancing these juicy texts within academic settings, I found many pissed and passionately poking holes in my eroticized homotextual gestures. As a nontenured visiting professor I was warned of the potentially terminal repercussions of sharing such leaky notions—potent concepts that were dangerously transformed as they flowed into dis-eased minds unwelcoming any sexual advances. In their resistance to the difficult knowledge (Britzman, 1998) of xenophobia, racist, classist, and (hetero)sexist theories infecting art education, I must ask myself if I had not properly aroused their curiosity before thrusting such naked truths into their minds.

> What I look for rather is a confrontational teaching of the humanities that would question the students' received disciplinary ideology (model of legitimate cultural explanations)...the unquestioned explicating power of the theorizing mind and class, the need for intelligibility and the rule of law... [A] pedagogy of the humanities as the arena of cultural explanations that questions the explanations of culture. (Spivak, 1990, p. 391)

If, as Marcuse (1978) asserts, the strength of art lies in its Otherness and its incapacity for ready assimilation, is it desirable, appropriate, or even possible to seduce students through discursive foreplay in order to prepare them to be penetrated by pedagogical practices, texts, art, and activists who talk sex? Are there ways to titillate yearnings for embracing the productivity of (dis)pleasure and still resist being held hostage to dominant discourses of safe sex as prohibition and abstinence, or art as useless, intentionally decorative, or simply containers of ideas? The unruly texts of artists open up fertile spaces of inquiry that I argue we must explore as educators. But in the context of cognitive contagion, how can we craft a conceptual condom that might ensure safe entry into socially dis-eased minds?

Cruising the Web for Visual Cultural Artifacts and Conceptual Condoms

Recognizing that intertextual analyses of visual and linguistic bodies always arouse my thinking, in the midnight hours I began cruising the Web for prophylactic representations—visual citations that might excite my discussion of visual culture, social dis-ease, and safer pedagogical practices. At first experiencing laughter, a bit of arousal, and a longing for a further deconstructive turn, these www. references reminded me of the uncomfortable self-knowledge that I'm still a size queen (the original tool rule peter meter, available at condomania.com). So to regain focus, I virtually donned my condom thinking cap (gagsplus.com) and soon realized I had not been thinking about sex safety as a branding concern or condoms as integral to consumptive identity. Knowing already that there were condoms in every flavor and color (prophylactics I imagine designed for devotees of Gardner's Multiple Intelligences [1983/1993]), I soon discovered I could purchase cultural celebratory condoms, from triple-pack snowman rubbers and mistletoe-labeled singles (though there were no Kwanzaa or Day of the Dead jimbos to be found) to studded Wrangler sheaths I was warned to have in "my back pocket before riding out into the sunset." From justrubbers.com I discovered I could purchase a "hot rod" condom that quickly applied itself, by simply pulling the appropriately placed tab in the heat of pleasure (Evelyn Wood's delight). The range of products, from gag bridal shower gifts of floral art (flower petals of wrapped rubbers) to KISS condoms (for the aging rocker), suggests I might need to be offering multiple conceptual prophylactic options for students, that is, if they are to safely enter group aesthetic intercourse.

There were also condom web sites that seemed yearning to be penetrated by Giroux's (1994a, 1994b) analyses of corporate product marketing—rubbers absolving consumer's guilt/inaction on political concerns as passions political and physical purportedly are addressed instantly by purchasing prescribed products (20 percent of all sales of Play Safe products at WACKY-JAC go to Tapestry Health). Finding these visual texts a turnoff, I continued manipulating my mouse, only to discover that my disinterest in sex could be easily accommodated if I took matters in my own hand and purchased the anti-intellectualist condom (pen for the academic dickhead). With visual titillations now considered, I return to an aesthetic examination of pedagogical prophylactics and the queer theoretical tricks such a challenge invites. I mount the challenge ready to rise to the occasion and aiming to emit a righteous load of provocative art initiatives that might entice the reader to join in the passionate work of critical visual cultural studies.

Fucking with Education History, Social Disease, and the Politically Promiscuous Artist

Progressive-era educators at the beginning of the twentieth century argued that child-centered and arts-based learning would excite students' curiosity and personal responsibilities in learning (Carhart, 1928; Malvern, 1995; Montessori, 1912; Steiner, 1923). These fertile cognitive theories, while embraced by myriad educators for their liberatory possibilities, can concurrently be framed as condoms for social dis-ease. Ross, in *Prophylactics Against Mob Mind*, asserted, "It is the concern of organized society to ...consider the various conditions that favor the growth of strong, robust individualities [as] proof against mental contagion" (1919). Dewey, in *Art as Experience* (1934), coupled intimate transformative encounters and methods of artists' inquiry with work-centered learning and practice of democratic values. WPA artist-activist-mounted social critiques (Lippard, 1999) are seldom studied in art/education programs today. Institutional challenges that were feared by politicians of the day later attracted the gaze of the House Committee on Un-American Activities. But war after war, interrupted by economic disaster (sound familiar?), convinced federal politicians that they needed to forcibly enter the educational womb of state, touting its desirability as a (re)productive space they could commandeer to stop the spread of rampant dis-ease over national security (the communist threat) and competitiveness.

Politicians' interest in education as a prophylactic against contagion capitalized on epidemic logic to produce a plethora of federal education legislation in the mid-twentieth century. Aroused by Sputnik in 1957, reform proponents begot the Education Defense Act of 1958; racial unrest, rural and urban poverty of the early 1960s begat the Elementary and Secondary Education Act of 1965; and feminist demands for gender equity birthed legislators' bastard child, Title IX. Meanwhile, as B. Ruby Rich (1994) notes, the many grass-roots liberation and power movements of the 1960s and '70s "opened space for enhanced participation...and inspired new forms of aesthetic inventions" (Becker, 1994, p. 226). So it seems while federal policy makers were raising their educational reform progeny, artists were dismounting their pedestals and hitting the streets, not seeking to avoid political penetration but undressing institutions and practices—taking them on publicly. Attacked "from a right-wing phalanx in need of a quick fix" (Becker, 1994, p. 226) in the wake of the Cold War, artists' institutional and social critiques were framed as pornographic and blasphemous. Artists responded with cries of First Amendment violations, but made little headway in the 1980s and early '90s. So in entering the political arena, NEA Chair Jane Alexander rolled on the trusty arts education prophylactic, parading school and community arts initiatives to diffuse the fluid transfer of dis-eased Reagan-era *Culture Wars* and the homophobic sputum of Senator Helms. At Clinton's pleasure, "Art" as the "fourth R" was added to Goals 2000 and the unfunded mandate was entered into law. But this seemingly sanctioned intercourse of interests aimed at satisfying a longing for a quality of educational experience that embraced the whole person, the arts, and the community was an affair of promise interrupted as the residents and priorities in the White House changed.

Change itself has been a passionate concern of artists in the last decades of the late twentieth century. That passion continues as product and message merge in postmodern artist-led social change initiatives, performing provocative interventions (Harper, 1998), which address multiple indentificatory possibilities (Gran Fury, Tim Miller, Guillermo Gómez-Peña, Coco Fusco, Rachel Rosenthal, James Luna), unleash the power potential of groups (Guerrilla Girls, Group Material, ACT UP), and construct institutional critiques (Andrea Fraser, Fred Wilson, Joyce Scott). The works of artists engaging in social change holds great potential for educators willing to (re)consider the ends of education. Recycling pedestals into barricades in the streets, these artists' discursive bodies have seductive appeal to educators willing to encounter the alterity of their texts, which invite them to enter into the fray of politics. Educators, administrators, and policy makers have largely ignored these politically alluring aesthetic actions, but such works are potentially productive in undressing socially provocative issues. Meaningfully incorporated into the school curriculum (Cahan & Kocur, 1996), such subjects stimulate students' awareness of critical social issues, disrupting their ambivalence and disinterest in schooling as a site of technological training and challenging them to take responsibility for creating a better world.

Visual cultural studies are valuable to educators unpacking media constructions of consumption and engaging students in practicing safer, more joyous, socially equitable, and sustainable ways of being in the world. Emerging from cultural studies (Dyer, 1992; Hall, 2001; Kellner, 1995; Marcuse, 1978; Williams, 1976), critical (Durham & Kellner, 2001; Friere, 1973; Giroux, 1994a; Lippard, 1990; McClaren, 1997), race and postcolonial (Bhabha, 1984; Gómez-Peña, 1994; Hawley, 2001; hooks, 1990, 1994, 1995; Trinh T. Minh-ha, 1989, 1991, 1992; West, 1994, 1995), semiotic (Barthes, 1998; Deleuze & Guattari, 1990), feminist (Britzman, 1998; Cixous, 1990; Garber, 1996; Gever, 1990; Spivak, 1990) and queer (Butler, 1997; Crimp & Rolston, 1990; D'Emilio, Turner, & Vaid, 2002, Duberman, 1997; Dyer, 1992; Foucault, 1985; Horne & Lewis, 1996; Jagose, 1996; Katz, 1976; Russo, 1987; Sanders, 2004; Saslow, 1999; Sedgwick, 1990; Somerville, 2000; Spargo, 1999; Wittig, 1990) theories exploring social behaviors and interactions, visual cultural studies in current art education literature (Ballangee-Morris & Stuhr, 2001; Carpenter, 1999; Duncum & Bracey, 2001; Efland, Freedman, & Stuhr, 1996; Freedman & Hernández, 1998; Jagodzinski, 1999) further simplify often critiqued elitist discourses of postmodern thought, calling for classroom educators to study and engage students in the rethinking of social possibilities through myriad visual texts.

Praxis of Visual Cultural Studies and the Rough Trade of Public Education

Visual cultural studies may be considered a way to explore social/cultural dynamics and meaning. How such studies are applied in entering the minds of student bodies is a slippery subject requiring conscious (pre)caution. Unlike the ample instructions provided with a studded condom, there is no printed direction for how to use the sheath of visual cultural studies as safe practice for students' liaisons with the provocative subjects artists potently portray. There are no guarantees that artists' leaky notions can be effectively shielded; thus educators wary of parental or administrative reprisals often opt for abstinence rather than be accused of making unwanted advances on students by requiring them to attend to artists' meanings. Insertion of visual cultural studies in teaching spaces before educators feel protected in passionately embracing the artists' concerns can be considered a dangerous practice. Tales of two such roughbacking educational encounters follow; the first exploring a cultural curriculum coordinator's condemnation of "risky" practices in an arts-in-education partnership, and the second examining an artist's indignation at a curator's refusal to expose students to her vaginal vessel's residual content.

Artists' representations of difference may be multiply intended, produced, and studied—at times in ways that can challenge K–12 students to consider webs of social regularities and cultural dynamics. In 1992, at the Southeastern Surface Design Association Symposium, *Cultural Foundations,* a gallery presentation of leading participants' works was mounted to explore the relationships between surface design and identity. The exhibit component was a central highlight of the sponsoring center's arts-in-education program, an artist-led, six-part unit for grades six to eight involving their viewing and study of relationships among visual patterns, ethnicity, and cultural identity. Of the seven artists, two were African-American, one Japanese, two Caucasian, one Latino, and one Native American. But what was at first not understood or appreciated was that the majority of these leaders were culturally self-identified as gay or bisexual.

All school teaching teams had completed in-service workshops that introduced links among patterning, design, and ethnic cultural identity—the big idea behind the unit—each enjoying hands-on practice in the art-making technologies (batik, block printing, photo-silk screening, and stenciling). No note was made, however, of the specific ways contemporary fiber artists were utilizing these techniques to broach a wide array of formal and social issues, as the exhibition itself had not been installed, nor its contents confirmed beyond the range of media/techniques of the exhibiting artists. The center's half-dozen teaching artists were already well underway with in-school slide-lectures for all 2,000 participating students as the exhibition was being hung. The first viewing of the exhibit by city/county schools' cultural and visual arts specialists took place at the symposium aligned with its opening, but only after the weekend's exciting series of workshops, lectures, and panel discussions did these school leaders come forth to articulate their concern, demanding the draping of two bodies of work they found offensive or insisting that students not be taken through the exhibit.

The "offending" exhibiting leader's art specifically grappled with representation of gay identity and AIDS. His contributions included a suite of manipulated Polaroid self-portraits that explored the pain he endured after a divorce judge homophobically decreed him unfit to see his children, and a pair of large pieces centrally portraying gay HIV+ friends at the prime of their health. Of the suite of head and upper torso Polaroid self-portraits, one depicted a dagger in the artist's heart, and its title alluded to the court case. Bordering each large image were seamlessly collaged Polaroid close-ups (none sexually explicit) of the subjects and their published obituary—texts noting the deceased's achievements and social involvements, but neither referencing AIDS. The artist's celebration of each subject's life served as a refutation of the demeaning practice of representing *victims* of the epidemic and conflations of gay identity with death, disease, and disgust. Alternately, textual silences contained in these obituaries call attention to the stigmatization and social dis-ease about an *unspeakable* pandemic.

The two cultural arts leaders from the school system admonished the center for not providing advance warning that such "controversial" images would be included in what they had assumed would be a *straight*forward presentation of multicultural art (i.e., craft of the Other). They asserted that to continue as planned with student gallery visits would jeopardize this or future arts-in-education partnerships and possibly result in the elimination of the schools' visual arts programs. They argued that neither artist-educators nor classroom teachers were qualified to discuss HIV/AIDS with middle-school students, and that trained health specialists, psychologists, and counselors were the only appropriate school staff to guide student discussion. They contended further that parents would have to be notified of the (potentially "offensive") content of the exhibit and offered an opportunity to exclude their children's participation in the exhibit visit. At the last minute, therefore, this revered exhibit (NEA/NEH, local and State Arts Councils awarded grants supporting the program) was determined a risk to be avoided or censored if children were to lay eyes on it.

Amidst the skirmishes still waging in the culture wars of the early 1990s, the center would not concede to acts of censorship, and further argued that *all* teachers should consider human rights, health, and dignity a subject of central importance in their teaching. Nonetheless, reading the exhibit as an ideologically infected body unfit for middle-school student embrace, school cultural arts leaders' compromise was to allow students to gaze on the exhibit only from the windows lining an exterior wall—a view rendering the "offending art" nearly invisible and most other works too distanced to touch their meaning. Lost was the opportunity to encounter the wide range of concerns the artists collectively raised—from contemporary adaptations of traditional Navajo symbolism in weaving; links among nationalism, terrorism, and Latino identity; or Japanese shiborri vessels as metaphors for Asian women's objectification; to Afrocentric silk paintings and enigmatic ritual garments made of urban refuse. But at what cost are some discourses entered while others are avoided like the plague?

A second dangerous liaison with visual cultural studies in this same Southeastern urban arts center involved not only fourth grade students across the county's schools but an artist whose work was accepted in a nationally juried exhibition of ceramics. In this arts-in-education program, students visited the "Common Ground" exhibition as part of a multilesson unit on pottery as a vessel for social and cultural meaning. The artist in question had submitted a wall-mounted clay sculpture, simply titled, but including a technique and materials description that read like an inventory of evidence from a crime scene. Before mounting the exhibit, the show's coordinator had determined that—rather than calling attention to the technologies involved in the creation of the multiple works—title, artist name, and date would consistently be entered on a wall-mounted identifying label. A catalog listing every work, with detailed technical data, was published with local corporate underwriting and given to every student visiting the exhibit. But fearing reprisals comparable to the earlier account, in every catalog given to elementary-age students, the coordinator carefully marked through the provocative work's material listing. The arts-in-education initiative proceeded without any protest from school partners or sponsor.

Even without any content listings, students (by this time numbering a thousand) had consistently cited the work in question as the "creepiest" and "scariest" in the show—many creating wildly imaginative stories as they interpreted and responded to works in the exhibit. Consisting of a single container with menacing tentacles, the work was powerful. A ceramic shrine to injustice, it documented the artist's experience as a victim of date-rape, its contents including the perpetrator's semen, K-Y Jelly, pubic hair and saliva—all specimens used in the court case. The artist (a college peer of the exhibit coordinator), learning of his resolution, deemed it a censoring of her work (although in this case, one not involving the actual removal or draping of the piece itself) and demanded that it be removed from the exhibit if the listing of contents within the vessel was not fully described on the wall label. The work was removed.

In both of these arts-in-education programs, overall curriculum design, school partnerships, grant funding, and sponsorship were secured well before the exhibitions were juried or curated. Should I consider consummating collaborations before applying visual cultural studies as a prophylactic a dangerous practice for which there are likely no guarantees? What contemporary art can we safely encounter with students if the body of the text is not known? Is a disorderly curricular courtship fatally flawed from its conception? How do fear of contagion or death of our arts-in-education programs result in a reluctance or refusal to engage unruly cultural texts?

Eric Rofes (1988) calls for working with school boards in motivating administrators and teachers' "effort[s] to stop AIDS in the United States" (p. 63). He notes that as a controversial subject, school administrators will more readily address such topics if supported by policies affecting huge numbers of children. Cahan and Kocur (1996), in *Contemporary Art and Multicultural Education*, detail HIV curriculum and lesson plans, describing the level of planning and preparation art teachers must undertake to safely enter the discursive spaces contemporary artists open up for their studies. Their twenty-five-lesson unit on HIV/AIDS draws on works from Gran Fury, David Wojnarowicz, and ACT UP (among others) to address the links among the pandemic, social injustice, and racist/sexist social practices.

Visual cultural studies currently in vogue in art education draw on media studies (Duncum & Bracey, 2001), film (Parks, 2004), and 1930s and '40s social reconstructionist art (Goetz-Zwirn, 2004)—from Jacob Lawrence (pp. 26–27), Dorothea Lange (28–29), and Ben Shawn (30–32) to comic books (Bitz, 2004, pp. 33–39)—to address race, class, and sexism but never broach the "Q" word or homophobia that seems so pervasive in media coverage of debates over partner benefits and same-sex marriage. It is telling that while popular discourse has been willing to redress social injustices around class, race, and feminist concerns of the past half-century, there is still little attention paid to the leading edge of social change surrounding same-sex relations.

Will it take art educators another fifty years before studying art that addresses civil rights for those whose relations deny heterosexual privilege? Is there currently a conceptual condom that can stand up to the religious right's puncturing perceptions of rough sex-talk about gay, lesbian, and transgendered couples relations? Is it possible for visual cultural studies to mount this challenge based on the current body of artistic and media texts? Or will educators need to continue cruising the Internet to excite their own strategies for marketing safer social-sexual practices in their teaching and conceptualization of curriculum?

While most are fearful of reprisals and often reluctant to take on socially relevant concerns, a few brave art educators do persist. Visual cultural studies as a provocative and productive practice can arouse students' imaginations, their passion for social change, and mastery of critical skills in undressing complex social issues. These practices should sheath educators as we penetrate discourses of contagion like No Child Left Behind, which renders student bodies and schools infected and in need of discipline and intervention. Cloaked in cultural studies condoms, we may more confidently tongue *Front Line*'s exposé on the culture of corporate tax evasion, or fuck with front-page images and headlines of politicians in drag as democratic warriors, repeatedly thrusting their hardened resolve to spread U.S. global capitalism into the well-oiled exotic Mideast.[1] Perhaps by wrapping ourselves in examinations of visual culture we can feel the dangerously throbbing political discourses thrust down our throats without swallowing their diseased messages.

Note

[1] Noam Chomsky, in his CBS interview on January 28, 2004, notes that the Bush administration's "domestic policies are...devastating to future generations. They're going have to pay the cost of this reactionary stateism where you have a huge state and you cut taxes for the wealthy....And the population doesn't like it, so you've got to get their mind off it, have to frighten them, you have to make them think that some demon's coming after them, so you have to huddle underneath the powerful leader who will protect you" (Noam Chomsky, interviewed by Evan Solomon, Canadian Broadcasting Corporation program *Hot Type* on January 28, 2004).

Bibliography

Ballangee-Morris, C., and Stuhr, P. (2001). Multicultural art and visual cultural education in a changing world. *Art Education, 54*(4): 6–13.

Barthes, R. (1998). Rhetoric of the image. In N. Mirzoeff (Ed.), *Visual culture reader*. New York: Routledge.

Becker, C. (Ed.). (1994). *The subversive imagination: Artists, society, and social responsibility*. New York: Routledge.

Bhabha, H. K. (1984). Representation and the colonial text. In F. Gloversmith (Ed.), *Theory of reading*. Sussex, U.K.: Harvester Press.

Bitz, M. (2004). The comic book project: The lives of urban youth. *Art Education: The Journal of the National Art Education Association, 57*(2). Reston, VA: NAEA.

Britzman, D. (1998). *Lost subjects, contested objects: Toward a psychoanalytic inquiry of learning*. Albany: State University of New York Press.

Butler, J. (1997). *The psychic life of power: Theories in subjection*. Stanford, CA: Stanford University Press.

Cahan, S., and Kocur, Z. (Eds.). (1996). *Contemporary art and multicultural education*. New York: New Museum of Contemporary Art and Routledge.

Carhart, A. H. (1928). Beauty and education. *School and Society,* 7 April, pp. 411–413.

Carpenter, S. (1999). Thoughts on black art and stereotypes: Visualizing racism. *Journal of Multicultural and Cross-cultural Research in Art Education, 17*: 103–115.

Cixous, H. (1990). Castration or decapitation? In R. Ferguson, M. Gever, M. Trinh, and C. West (Eds.), *Out there: Marginalization and contemporary cultures* (pp. 345–356). Cambridge, MA: New Museum of Contemporary Art & Massachusetts Institute of Technology Press.

Crimp, D., and Rolston, A. (1990). *AIDS demographics.* Seattle, WA: Bay Press.

Deleuze, G. and Guattari, F. (1990). What is a minor literature? In R. Ferguson, M. Gever, M. Trinh, and C. West (Eds.), *Out there: Marginalization and contemporary cultures* (pp. 59–70). Cambridge, MA: New Museum of Contemporary Art & Massachusetts Institute of Technology Press.

D'Emilio, J., Turner, W. B., and Vaid, U. (Eds.). (2002). *Creating change: Sexuality, public policy, and civil rights.* New York: St. Martin's Press.

Dewey, J. (1934/1980). *Art as experience.* New York: Perigee Books.

Duberman, M. (Ed.). (1997). *Queer representations: Reading lives, reading cultures: A center for lesbian and gay studies book.* New York and London: New York University Press.

Duncum, P., and Bracey, T. (Eds.). (2001). *On knowing: Art and visual culture.* Christchurch, New Zealand: Canterbury Press.

Durham, M., and Kellner, D. M. (Eds.). (2001). *Media and cultural studies: Keyworks.* Malden, MA: Blackwell Publishers.

Dyer, R. (1992). *Only entertainment.* New York: Routledge.

Efland, A., Freedman, K., and Stuhr, P. (1996). *Postmodern art education: An approach to curriculum.* Reston, VA: The National Art Education Association.

Foucault, M. (1985). *The uses of pleasure.* New York: Pantheon.

Freedman, K., and Hernández, F. (Eds.). (1998). *Curriculum, culture, and art education: Comparative perspectives.* Albany: State University of New York Press.

Friere, P. (1973/1998). *Education for critical consciousness.* New York: Continuum Publishing.

Garber, E. (1996). Art criticism from a feminist point of view: An approach for teachers. In G. Collins and R. Sandell (Eds.), *Gender issues in art education: Content, contexts and strategies.* Reston, VA: National Art Education Association.

Gardner, H. (1993). *Frames of mind: The theory of multiple intelligences* (10th anniversary edition). New York: Basic Books.

Gever, M. (1990). The names we give ourselves. In R. Ferguson, M. Gever, M. Trinh, and C. West (Eds.), *Out there: Marginalization and contemporary cultures* (pp. 191–202). Cambridge, MA: New Museum of Contemporary Art & Massachusetts Institute of Technology Press.

Giroux, H. A. (1994a). *Disturbing pleasures: Learning popular culture.* New York: Routledge.

———. (1994b). Benetton's 'World Without Borders': Buying social change. In Carol Becker (Ed.), *The subversive imagination: Artists, society, and social responsibility* (pp. 187–207). New York: Routledge.

Goetz-Zwirn, S. (2004). Men and women at work: The portrayal of American workers by three artists of the 1930s and 1940s. *Art Education, 57*(2): 25–32.

Gómez-Peña, G. (1994). Hybrid America. In A. Patner (Ed.), *Alternative futures: Challenging designs for arts philanthropy* (pp. 80–88). Philadelphia: Grantmakers in the Arts.

Hall, S. (2001). Encoding/decoding. In M. G. Durham and D. Kellner (Eds.), *Media and cultural studies: Keyworks* (pp. 177–197). Malden, MA: Blackwell Publishers.

Harper, G. (Ed.). (1998). *Interventions and provocations: Conversations on art, culture, and resistance.* Albany: State University of New York Press.

Hawley, J. C. (Ed.). (2001). *Postcolonial, queer: Theoretical intersections.* Albany: State University of New York Press.

hooks, b. (1990). *Yearnings: Race, gender, and cultural politics.* Boston: South End Press.

———. (1994). *Outlaw culture: Resisting representation.* New York: Routledge.

———. (1995). *Art on my mind: Visual politics.* New York: The New Press.

Horne, P., and Lewis, R. (Eds.). (1996). *Outlooks: Lesbian and gay sexualities and visual cultures.* New York: Routledge.

Jagodzinski, J. (1999). Reading Hollywood's post-racism: Lessons for art education. *Journal of Multicultural and Cross-cultural Research in Art Education,* 17: 74–90.

Jagose, A. (1996). *Queer theory: An introduction.* New York: New York University Press.

Katz, J. (1976). *Gay American history: Lesbians and gay men in the U.S.A.: A documentary history.* New York: Thomas Y. Crowell Company.

Kellner, D. (1995). *Media culture: Cultural studies, identity, and politics between the modern and the postmodern.* New York: Routledge.

Lippard, L. (1990). *Mixed blessings: New art in a multicultural America.* New York: Pantheon.

———. (1999). In B. Wallis, M. Weems, and P. Yenawine (Eds.), *Art matters: How the culture wars changed America.* New York: NYU Press.

Malvern, S. B. (1995). Inventing 'child': Franz Cizek and modernism. *The British Journal of Aesthetics,* 35: 262–272.

Marcuse, H. (1978). *The aesthetic dimension.* Boston: Beacon Press.

McLaren, P. (1997). *Revolutionary multiculturalism: Pedagogies of dissent for the new millennium*. Boulder, CO: Westview Press.

Montessori, M. (1912). The Montessori method; Scientific pedagogy as applied to child education. In A. E. George (trans.), *The children's houses*. New York: Frederick A. Stokes.

Parks, N. S. (2004). Bamboozled: A visual culture text for looking at cultural practices of racism. *Art Education, 57*(2): 14–18.

Rich, B. R. (1994). Dissed and disconnected. In C. Becker (Ed.), *The subversive imagination: Artists, society, and social responsibility*. New York: Routledge.

Rofes, E. (1988). Working with your local school board. In S. Alyson (Ed.), *You can do something about AIDS* (pp. 63–64). Boston: The Stop AIDS Project.

Ross, E. A. (1919). Prophylactics against mob mind. *Social psychology: An outline and source book* (pp. 83–93). New York: Macmillan Co.

Russo, V. (1987). *The celluloid closet: Homosexuality in the movies* (revised edition). New York: Harper & Row.

Sanders, J. (2004). Moving beyond the binary. In A. Fariello and P. Owen (Eds.), *Objects and meaning: Readings that challenge the norm*. Lanham, MD: Scarecrow Press.

Saslow, J. M. (Ed.). (1999). *Pictures and passions: A history of homosexuality in the visual arts*. New York: Penguin Books.

Sedgwick, E. K. (1990). *Epistemology of the closet*. Los Angeles: University of California Press.

Singer, L. (1993). *Erotic welfare: Sexual theory and politics in the age of epidemic*. New York: Routledge.

Somerville, S. B. (2000). *Queering the color line: Race and the invention of homosexuality in American culture.* Durham, NC and London: Duke University Press.

Spargo, T. (1999) *Postmodern encounters: Foucault and queer theory.* New York: Totem Books USA.

Spivak, G. C. (1990). Explanation and culture: Marginalia. In R. Ferguson, M. Gever, M. Trinh, and C. West (Eds.), *Out there: Marginalization and contemporary cultures* (pp. 377–394). Cambridge, MA: New Museum of Contemporary Art & Massachusetts Institute of Technology Press.

Steiner, R. (1923/1964). *The arts and their mission.* Eight lectures delivered in Dornach, Switzerland, May 27–June 9, 1923, and in Kristiana (Oslo), Norway, May 18 and 20, 1923. Translation by Lisa D. Monges and Virginia Moore. New York: Anthroposophic Press.

Trinh, M. (1989). *Woman, native, other: Writing postcoloniality and feminism.* Bloomington: Indiana University Press.

———. (1991). *When the moon waxes red: Representation, gender, and cultural politics.* New York: Routledge.

———. (1992). *Framer framed.* New York: Routledge.

West, C. (1994). *Race matters.* New York: Vintage Books.

———. (1990). The new cultural politics of difference. In R. Ferguson, M. Gever, M. Trinh, and C. West (Eds.), *Out there: Marginalization and contemporary cultures* (pp. 19–38). Cambridge, MA: New Museum of Contemporary Art & Massachusetts Institute of Technology Press.

Williams, R. (1976). *Keywords: A vocabulary of culture and society.* New York: Oxford University Press.

Wittig, M. (1990). The straight mind. In R. Ferguson, M. Gever, M. Trinh, and C. West (Eds.), *Out there: Marginalization and contemporary cul-*

tures (pp. 51–58). Cambridge, MA: New Museum of Contemporary Art & Massachusetts Institute of Technology Press.

• CHAPTER SEVEN •

Condoms, Penis Size, and Statistics:
One Size Definitely Does Not Fit All!

Michael J. Nanna

I'm not sure where to find the source exactly, but somewhere I learned that the average adult male penis size is 6 inches in length. It was data that I probably obtained from reading one of the alternative "academic" journals that are on the market. Although there is no doubt legitimate data on both penis length and width, I was afraid to look. Chalk it up to one of those silly nonfunctional heterosexual hang-ups. You know, the ones that us liberal types deny we have. However, given the challenge of writing this chapter, which has as its focus a "statistical" analysis of penis size in relationship to available condom sizes, I started poking around for the needed empirical data. To my surprise, I found an abundance of available secondary data (though finding an original source proved difficult). For example, according to a 1950s report from the Alfred C. Kinsey Institute for Sex, the average erect penis length for white college men was 6.16 inches in length, with a girth of 4.84 inches.[1] (www.edu.uni-klu.ac.at/~amiklaut/dr_nick/answer19.htm). Moreover, according to a study by Ansell Limited, makers of Life-Styles Condoms, a research study investigating average penis size found the average length of the erect penis to be 5.877 (SD = 0.825; n = 300) inches, with the majority of penises ranging between 5.5 and 6.3 inches in length. The study also found the average girth to be roughly 4.972 inches (SD = 0.508) with the majority ranging between 4.7 and 5.1 inches in circumference (www.free-condom-stuff.com/fcs/html/penis-average-size.html). Finally, a study by Durex found the average length to be 6.4 inches, with an average width of 5.2 inches at the widest part (www.pridepenis.co.uk/What is the average size of a penis.htm).

Although the Durex study did contain data from multiple countries, none of the studies categorized data by ethnicity, so I'll just assume that—although the average penis size may vary across racial and ethnic categories—the variation is homogeneous across groups and that there is sufficient overlap in the possible distributions to warrant some degree of generalization. In statistical terms: There may be an acknowledged shift in location parameter between groups without subsequent change in spread or variation (i.e., homogeneity of variance). For the purposes of this "study," in order to estimate the average penis size of all men in...well...the world, I decided to take the average of the three studies mentioned above. This resulted in an average estimated penis size of roughly 6.15 inches. For simplicity and ease of calculation, I decided to round the average down to 6 inches.

Before beginning, I would like to make explicit several assumptions about penis size for the purposes of this study. First, let's assume that penis size, like many naturally occurring variables, tends toward a normal distribution, that is, the distribution of penis size varies naturally, which means that if we were to plot all penis sizes on a frequency distribution, the shape of the resulting distribution would resemble a normal distribution, or bell curve. Remember that word? In fact, the data from the Kinsey study outlined above found just that[2]:

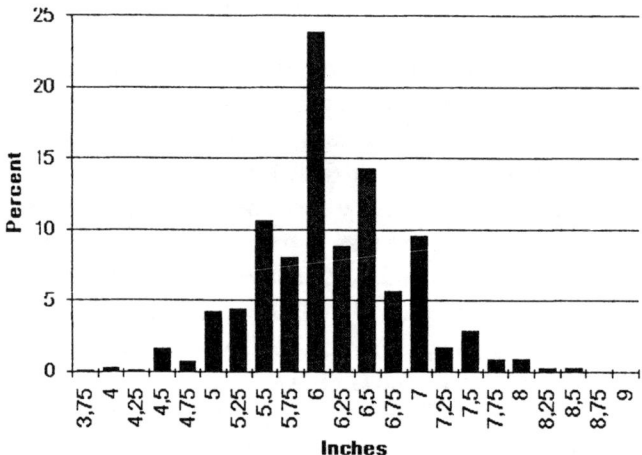

I guess a lot of things that I never thought of as following a bell curve actually do. At least, so we've been told by Herrnstein and Murray (1994). Of course, this study is probably more biased and less accurate than theirs, but at least in this case we have access to "hard" data (pun definitely intended!).

And Now Back to Penis Size
I have already established that the average male penis size is roughly equal to six inches in length. That means that if we were to collect data on the entire population of human males (presumably over the age of eighteen) and sum all of their penis sizes together and then divide by the total population size

(N), we would arrive at the actual population parameter, which in this case is symbolized by the Greek letter μ (pronounced mu). Thus, μ = 6". Having established one of the location parameters (in this case the mean) for the human male penis, we'll now turn to the variation. Here's where we'll have to use a little imagination. Let's assume[3] that the male penis has a standard deviation of 0.5 inches. Thus, σ = 0.5". That means that if we were to again look at our frequency distribution of scores of all human penises in the world (over the age of eighteen), most penises, in fact roughly 68 percent of them, would fall within -1.00 and +1.00 standard deviations about the mean. Thus, 68 percent of the world's penises are between 5.5 and 6.5 inches long. Further, roughly 98 percent of the world's penises would be between -2.00 and +2.00 standard deviations around the mean, which means that roughly 98 percent of the world's penises would fall between 5 and 7 inches in length. And finally, roughly 99 percent of the world's penises would fall between -3.00 and +3.00 standard deviations around the mean, resulting in 99 percent of the world's penises falling between 4.5 inches and 7.5 inches in length. A cursory examination of the table above will confirm that this seems to be the case, although penises in the Kinsey study ranged from 3.75 inches in length (poor fellows) and 9 inches in length (poor ladies). Keep in mind that I did "massage" the data for ease of calculation and pedagogical clarity, so the results are probably more congruent with the tabled Kinsey report results than my example suggests. Confused yet? Let's see if I can clear this up a bit with several working examples. Before working through an example, however, you'll first need a brief introduction to the normal distribution and continuous random variables.

Continuous Random Variables
A continuous random variable is a variable that can take on any value in an interval of numbers. For example, although we've established that the adult penis can vary in length, that variation is certainly not limited to ½-inch increments. The length of the human penis, being a continuous random variable, can take on an infinite number of measurements, depending only on the accuracy and sensitivity of our instrument. We could, if we wanted to do so, measure the human penis in nanometers; very small incremental units indeed.[4] Next, the probabilities associated with a continuous random variable (we'll call it "x" for the time being) are determined by the probability density function of the random variable. The function denoted f(x) has the following properties:

1. $f(x) \geq 0$ for x.
2. The probability that x will be between two numbers "a" and "b" is equal to the area under f(x) between "a" and "b."
3. The total area under the entire curve of f(x) is equal to 1.00.

Stated more succinctly (and in English), continuous random variables can take on an infinite number of values. Also, try to remember that probabilities range from 0 (no probability) to 1.00 (absolute certainty). Are you still with me? I didn't think so, but I'll continue anyway.

If we look at a normally distributed distribution of penis sizes and I ask you, "What is the probability of randomly selecting one penis size from that distribution?" what would your answer be? It should be 1.00, because all penis sizes are represented in the distribution. Now, let's say I ask you, "What is the probability of selecting a penis size that falls within some range; say between 3 and 6 inches?" In this case, the probability would be equal to the proportion of area on the distribution curve that lay between these two penis sizes. To provide some background to the problem, let's look at several characteristics of the normal distribution: (1) it's bell shaped (the mean, median, and mode are all equal), (2) it's symmetric about the mean (half of the values fall below the mean and the other half fall above the mean), and (3) it's completely described by the mean and standard deviation.

The z-Distribution
The z-distribution is a theoretical distribution also known as the standard normal distribution. The z-distribution allows us to standardize any variable that naturally follows, or tends toward, a normal distribution. The z-distribution has two primary qualities. First, it has a mean of 0 and a standard deviation of one. Z-scores are also known as standard deviation units. We can standardize any variable or score so long as we know both the population mean and standard deviation. This allows us to express differences in scores in standard deviation units.

Knowing that all of the area under the z-distribution (bell curve) is equal to 1.00 allows us to divide the distribution into equal units. For example, if I were interested in identifying the location on the distribution that would cut off the lower 2.5 percent and the upper 2.5 percent, all I would have to do is find a z-table (available in any introductory statistics book) and identify the z-score that cuts off the both the upper and lower 2.5 percent area of the curve (or .025 of the area). In this case, the z-values of -1.96 and + 1.96 are the z-scores that correspond to the place on the normal curve that cuts off the upper and lower 2.5 percent of the total area under the curve. The importance of these values will soon be evident.

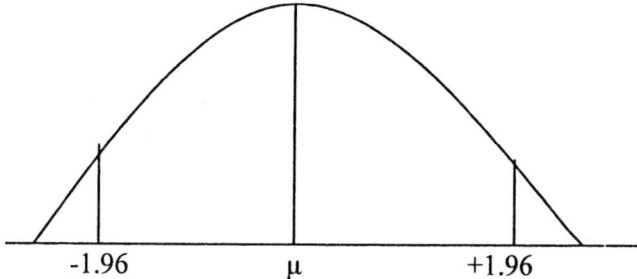

That means that 95 percent of the area of the normal curve falls between 1.96 and +1.96. Remember that every normal distribution (in this case the distribution of penis sizes) can be standardized using the following formula:

$$Z = \frac{X - \mu}{\sigma}$$

So let's start applying what we've learned thus far with an example.

Let's say that Julie knows that the average male adult penis is 6 inches in length with a standard deviation of 0.5 inches. What is the probability that a romantic encounter with a new partner will be with someone who has a penis size between 6 and 7 inches in length? You might be wondering why this is important. Well, for several reasons. First, Julie has to plan for the evening. I mean, she can't just be jumping into the sack with anyone without using protection, at least not in this day and age. So she has to be prepared with the appropriate protection against the plethora of sexually transmitted diseases currently on the "market," not to mention birth control (provided she's not currently taking oral contraceptives). Moreover, being a rather petite gal, she has to estimate the probability of whether or not her new partner's penis will fit comfortably inside her average-sized vagina. Most importantly, she has to somehow be sure that if they decide to use a condom, it will fit properly, which as we shall see, may prove more difficult than you might now imagine. Not so unimportant after all, is it? Do you see the potential discomfort that could be avoided with a little homework prior to a new sexual encounter? Finally, a "real life" use for statistics! Now back to the problem. I will give you a hint to the solution: We need to find the area under the curve between the corresponding z-values of 6 and 7 inches. Remember that 50 percent of the total area of the standard normal (z) distribution lies above the mean, and 50 percent of the total area lies below the mean (that's that symmetric thing). So we know the following information:

µ = 6" (this is the mean, or estimated average penis size in the population)
σ = 0.5" (this is our estimated standard deviation of penis size in the population)
X = 7"

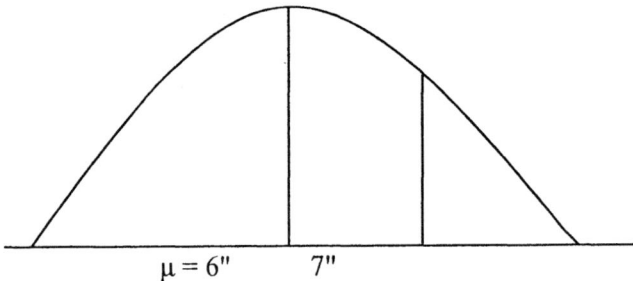

Therefore, using a simple z-formula, we get:

$$Z = \frac{X - \mu}{\sigma} = \frac{7" - 6"}{0.5"} = z = 2.00$$

We now have to find the area of the curve that lies between the mean (6") and our z-score for 7" (z = 2.00) by using the z-table. Ultimately, we are interested in estimating the probability of Julie finding a new sexual partner who has a penis size that falls somewhere between the mean (6") and two standard deviations above the mean, which in this case is 7", since the standard deviation is equal to 0.5" (2 * 0.5" = 1"). Got it?

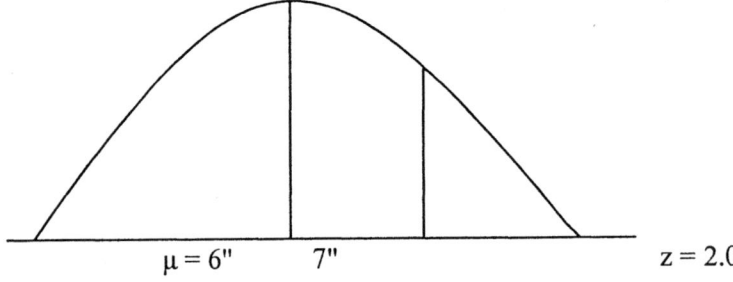

So looking at a z-table, we need to find the area that falls between the mean and our obtained z-score (+2.00). In this case, the area is equal to 0.4772 (or close to it). Therefore the answer to our question is that there is an almost 48 percent chance that Julie's new partner will have a penis size between 6 and 7 inches in length. Pretty good odds, if you ask me. But that also implies that there is a 52 percent chance that her new partner's penis is either shorter than six inches or longer than seven inches. The problem this may pose will present itself shortly. Or maybe it would be better to just say, soon!

Let's try another example, just to make sure that you understand the problem. What is the probability that Julie's new partner will have a penis size between 5 and 7 inches in length? Essentially we need to repeat the steps we just did, except this time we have to find the area between the mean and obtained z-value for the area both below the mean and above the mean. Then we merely add these two values together.

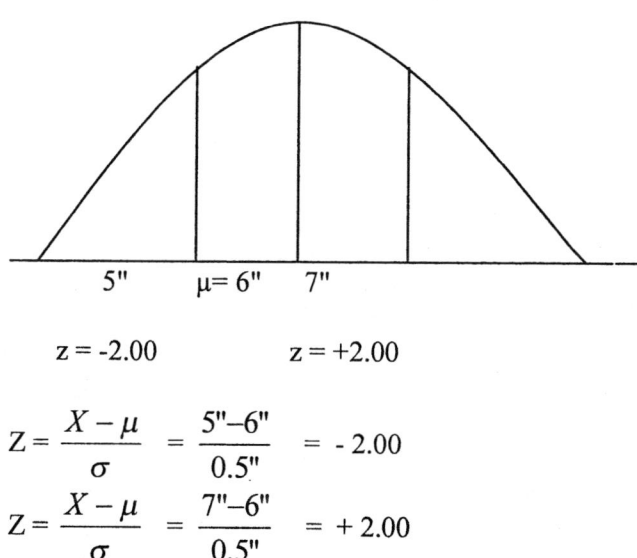

$$Z = \frac{X - \mu}{\sigma} = \frac{5''-6''}{0.5''} = -2.00$$

$$Z = \frac{X - \mu}{\sigma} = \frac{7''-6''}{0.5''} = +2.00$$

In this case we get an area of 0.4772 (z = -2.00) + 0.4772 (z = +2.00) = 0.9544. Therefore, there is a 95 percent chance that Julie's new partner will have a penis size between 5 and 7 inches in length. This information, as you may now see, is fairly important to Julie lest she risk serious injury, discomfort, exposure to sexually transmitted diseases, or, at the very least, waste money on condoms that don't fit—a problem that is more widespread than most people think.

Condoms Must Be Made to Fit Like a Glove

It occurred to me that given the variability of the adult penis size and the apparent narrow selection of available condoms on the market—most of which cater to the average penis length—many individuals may be unable to find an appropriately fitting condom. Condoms traditionally come in pre-determined sizes and vary only slightly between brands and styles. In fact, the distribution of condom sizes is not a continuous random variable tending toward a normal distribution at all, but rather one that resembles more of a uniform distribution.[5] If penis size does indeed vary in length and is distributed normally with a standard deviation of 0.5 to 1 inch, that means that there are quite a few people out there who may have trouble finding a properly fitting condom. The consequences should be obvious and are potentially devastating. For example, according to a source at www.the-penis-website.com/condom.html, "the number one reason that condoms break or slip off during lovemaking is that the penis in question was wearing the wrong size of condom." Moreover, according to the same web site, another study (though undocumented in this web site) found that nearly half of 3,000 survey respondents felt that the condoms they regularly used did not fit properly. Additional results suggest that 25 percent of the respondents claimed that their condoms were too tight, 10 percent said they were much too tight, and almost 7 percent said that the condoms were too loose or much too loose. The study concluded, "Given the wide range of penis sizes and the relatively narrow range of condoms designed to fit them, it is perhaps unsurprising to find that 50% of respondents felt that the condoms they used did not fit them properly." According to this same source, another study conducted by La Trobe University in Australia confirmed that penis size is related to condom breakage or slippage. The study included a total of 3,658 condoms used by 184 men. Over the course of the study, 16 percent of the men experienced at least one instance of breakage and 19 percent experienced complete slippage. So what, you ask? In addition to the obvious increased risk of pregnancy and exposure to sexually transmitted infections (STIs) I offer the following case study from a medical journal in India:

> A 27-year-old lady presented with persistent cough, sputum and fever for the preceding six months. In spite of trials with antibiotics and anti-tuberculosis treatment for the preceding four months, her symptoms did not improve. A subsequent chest radiograph showed non-homogeneous collapse-consolidation of right upper lobe. Video-bronchoscopy revealed an inverted baglike structure in right upper lobe bronchus and rigid bronchoscopic removal with biopsy forceps confirmed the presence of a condom. Detailed retrospective history also confirmed accidental inhalation of

the condom during fellatio (Arya, Gupta, & Arora, 2004).

It seems that the lack of appropriate condom sizes clearly presents a serious health risk beyond sexually transmitted infections and/or unintended pregnancy. Indeed, it would appear that this situation could have been avoided if only there had there been a more varied selection of condoms available on the market (at least in India), and the gentleman in question had been wearing a condom that fit properly. The best analogy I can think of is trying to fit a size six foot that has been lathered in petroleum jelly into a size ten shoe and then attempting to kick a field goal. Risk of slippage: high.

Measuring Up
So just how widespread is the problem of poorly fitting condoms? Although I don't have any large-scale epidemiological evidence in hand (or should I say, available), I think another illustrative (and theoretical) example will provide some clarity as to how common this problem may actually be. This time, instead of determining the probability of Julie having a sexual partner with a penis size that falls within a certain range, let's determine the lower and upper bounds of what could be considered the normal or standard penis size. Let's assume that the acceptable average penis size that can fit snugly into a standard condom falls between -1.00 and +1.00 standard deviations about the mean. Knowing what we know about our hypothetical average penis size and the standard deviation of our population, this suggests a penis that is between 5.5 and 6.5 inches schlong. I mean, long. For cost effectiveness and production efficiency alone, most condom manufacturers probably play the odds and manufacture condoms that cater to the average penis size; to do otherwise from a production standpoint would not be very cost-effective. But what of the probability that someone will have a penis size smaller than 5.5 inches or larger than 6.5 inches? Back to our normal distribution:

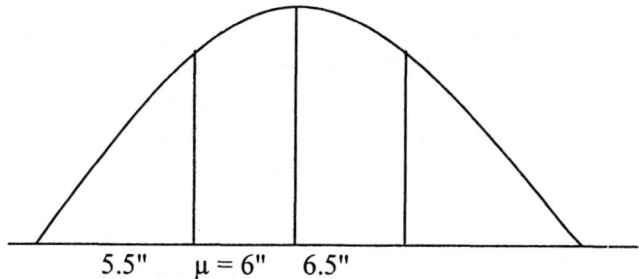

$$z = -1.00 \qquad z = +1.00$$

$$Z = \frac{X - \mu}{\sigma} = \frac{5.5'' - 6''}{0.5''} = -1.00$$

$$Z = \frac{X - \mu}{\sigma} = \frac{6.5'' - 6''}{0.5''} = +1.00$$

This time, instead of finding the area between the mean and our obtained z-score in a z-table, we want to determine the area of the curve that lies beyond our obtained z-values. Here we find that the area beyond a z-score of either 1.00 or +1.00 is equal to 0.1587, for a total area of 0.3174. That means that almost 32 percent of the adult male population is estimated to have a penis size that falls outside the normal bounds and is either too small or too big by standard definitions (ultimately, the terms "too big" or "too small" are relative, of course). In Vegas, those are damn good odds! The figure of 32 percent represents a significant portion of the male population, so you can see just how important this study really is. Condoms that are too small risk breaking mid-coitus and condoms that are too big risk...well...being inhaled. If that isn't a serious public health risk, then I don't know what is. Also, keep in mind that we've been talking only of length. Width is also an important indicator of condom fit, and given that condoms are also sized to fit width as well as length, deviations in girth might also prove problematic. However, I'll have to save the issue of girth for another study.

Lest you think it is just people from India who are at risk, I offer the following evidence. According to an article by Getzlaff (2000) that outlines a study conducted by Focus (presumably a market research firm in Europe) that cites a study conducted by the German condom manufacturer Condomi...(Do you see where this is going? Internet sources just don't adhere to rigorous citation standards that we in academia do). Anyway, whichever study it actually was, the study found that the standard European condom "fell off half of the men polled" (I know there's a joke in here somewhere!). More importantly, the study revealed that the size of the average German penis is about 3.5 to 4.0 millimeters (that's 0.13 to 0.15 inches for us English and American types) too narrow for the standard European (the EN600...sounds high tech) condom. According to Getzlaff (2000), "size really does matter." So are European men less endowed than their American counterparts? Although anecdotally I have heard that penis size does vary somewhat by ethnicity, it's not likely. Instead, it appears that the issue lay with the European condom itself. It seems that in 1996 the European Union decided to standardize the size of the European condom to 6.63 inches in length, with an acceptable width ranging from 1.7 to 2.2 inches (Getzlaff, 2000). Perhaps the condom makers in Europe were suffering from a little wishful thinking? Or maybe they relied on self-report studies when doing the market research. In any case, the size issue is complicated. Not only do we have to worry about appropriate length, we have to worry about width as well. Taking into account only one variable may prove to be shortsighted. Indeed, this means that finding a condom that fits the length of a penis is only half the battle, for a condom that fits lengthwise but not widthwise is sure to slip off. I must admit that prior to being invited to write this chapter I had never given much thought to the issue. I guess I must fall somewhere in the "normal" range (upper end of the distribution, of course). Still, the fact remains that in both the United States and Europe, condoms have been manufactured to meet the needs of the many, while ignoring the needs of the few.

The Taylor-Made Condom
Standardization is nothing new. In fact, it dates back to the early part of the twentieth century, when businesses were confronted with the need for a more efficient means of production. The pressures to standardize most likely stem from economic factors such as the need to control costs while maximizing both output and profit. It's easy to see why condoms have generally come in only one or two sizes. There wasn't much discussion regarding penis size until the Kinsey reports of the 1950s, so manufacturers probably just took a best guess. And given that there is often a lag time between new scientific information and widespread production and distribution of products, it's understandable why condoms have not come in more than a couple of sizes. It's marketing to the masses…to the average…to the 6-inchers. Standardization may have its strong points, but the data examined in this paper suggest that there is a large segment of the population that is excluded and discriminated against through the process of standardization. But no more! It turns out that there is hope for the world's off-size penises—be they too big or too small. Yes, Mr. Frederick Taylor, you can now officially roll over in your grave, because customization is the new wave of the future. Standardization is out and customization is in! Well, at least for condom sizes, as it appears that we have finally started to emerge from the dark ages of standardization, and leading the way is condom development. We can only hope that the trend

continues and leaks over into education, health care, and the fast-food industry.

Condom manufacturer *Condomania* has introduced the world's first sized-to-fit condoms, offering fifty-five—yes, fifty-five—custom-fitted condoms catering to nearly every penis length/width configuration. The promotional web site for *Condomania* claims that the benefits of wearing a properly fitting condom include increased pleasure and comfort as well as increased safety and reliability. Yes, kids, for the first time ever, you can shop for condoms just like you shop for clothing and shoes (www.condomania.com). The manufacturer notes,

> Of course, comfort is what consumers will notice most of all about They-Fit Condoms. A custom "wrap" job for each man begins with the simple "Fit Kit," which can be downloaded from *Condomania*'s Web site. The "Fit Kit" enables a man (or even his enthusiastic partner) to quickly and easily measure his penis length and girth according to the Fit Kit's proprietary sizing chart, which then displays the appropriate custom condom size. The dozens of available sizes ensure that men of all shapes and sizes will be able to be dressed properly for their big events. Men need not worry how they measure up with the "Fit Kit"; the proprietary numbering system is not relative to actual size. Thus ordering a box of B88s is no more embarrassing than ordering a box of Z11s. According to Sadlo, "It is important to note that these numbers are not relative to other letters and numbers, so that no one will be self-conscious about the size of the They Fit Condom they buy."

Not only can men around the world procure custom-fitted condoms, but they don't have to worry about the embarrassment associated with ordering a "less than average" sized condom. Yes, it's comfort, fit, and confidentiality all in one small (or large) package! According to a spokesperson from *Condomania*, this new line of custom-fit condoms represents the "biggest technological advance in condoms in a generation" (personal communication, March 11, 2004). Indeed!

Skewing the Results
It seems there is a glimmer of hope for all those unfortunate men whose "old fellas" fall outside "normal" limits. And just in time, as the largest evolutionary shift in average penis size is upon us. Indeed, an evolutionary process that would have Charles Darwin running for the hills. Several months ago I fell asleep watching what will remain an unnamed cable channel that caters to shows of a comedic nature (though it was most likely local programming). I awoke several times after 3 A.M. and remained in a state of reverie while listening to an endless (and mind-numbing) onslaught of infomercials di-

rected toward increasing one's penis size. In one of them, a much-too-happy female spokesmodel and her less-than-attractive male co-host/stooge spent an hour introducing a cadre of testimonials and professional endorsements from an expansive list of individuals that included urologists and even the local chiropractor. I watched dazed and half asleep as testimonial after testimonial professed ad nauseum the astounding benefits of the latest penis enlargement product—in this case, an easily digestible (and affordable!) pill. It seems that a larger and more robust penis is just several tablets away. Three o'clock in the morning must be the witching hour for infomercials, as this particular advertisement (or one similar to it) could be found on multiple stations; yes, penis TV. I guess the folks in market research determined that quite a few inadequately endowed men watch television into the wee hours. So I guess the old adage and 1970s liberal mantra that "size doesn't matter" has been co-opted by a new one: not only does size matter, it's the only thing that matters! How American. Now we can supersize our penises along with our value meals. Of course, the penis media blitz isn't limited to television. No, sir. A quick check of your e-mail inbox will most likely verify this. I offer the following excerpt from one of the dozens of e-mail SPAMS I receive on a daily…no…hourly basis as evidence:

* *No Pumps! No Surgery! No Exercises!*
* *NO.1 Penis Enlargement Pill on the Market!*
* *Gain 3+ Full Inches in Length*
* *Expand Your Penis Up to 20% Thicker*
* *Stop Premature Ejaculation!*
* *Produce Stronger Erections*
* *100% Safe to Take, with No Side Effects*

An increase of three full inches! That would increase the average human penis size significantly; to nine inches, in fact. Ouch. Dr. Frankenstein would certainly be proud, but messing with nature seems a bit dangerous, don't you think? I can only think of the 1980s B-movie *The Re-Animator*. What if these Frankensteinian penises came alive and began to think for themselves?[6] It is a scary scenario indeed. Not to mention the potential public health risk that so many unprotected penises would pose to society: sexually transmitted diseases; unintended pregnancy; inhalation! Thankfully we have no need to worry about such a monstrous occurrence; no need to worry about millions of unsheathed, conscious, nine-inch penises running wild in the streets ready for action without any available properly fitting condoms. *Condomania*'s deluxe line of custom-fit condoms will help to restrain this burgeoning population of nine-inch monster penises. Thanks to *Condomania*, we're covered (okay, pun intended that time).

Changing Seasons of the Condom
Condom use most likely dates back to ancient times. Images from about 1000 B.C. depict ancient Egyptians wearing linen sheaths, and early evidence from around A.D. 100 to 200 suggests that men in Europe used condoms frequently. In the 1500s in Italy, research by Gabrielle Fallopius discovered that the linen sheath was useful for prevention of infection, and that later the condom proved useful for the prevention of pregnancy. By 1844, the first mass-produced condoms were made available by Goodyear and Hancock, and were made out of vulcanized rubber—a stronger and more elastic material. Perhaps this is where the term "rubber" has its origin. I guess it's better than linen. By 1880 the first latex condom was produced, even though it wasn't until the 1930s that they were widely used.

Though developments in condom technology have followed a somewhat linear progression, condom use in the United States has not. In fact, it has ebbed and flowed with the times, frequently being affected by social and cultural trends. For example, in the early 1900s, some social hygienists attempted to prohibit the use of condoms by Americans. Unfortunately, propaganda aimed at prohibition of condom use resulted in U.S. troops during World War I having a very high rate of STDs. Luckily, by World War II temperance and condom sense—oops, I mean common sense—had prevailed as the U.S. government aggressively promoted the use of condoms to prevent pregnancy and the transmission of sexually transmitted diseases. But, as the sexual revolution of the 1960s loomed, condom use once again dipped with the advent of "free love" and the birth control pill (www.lifestyles.com/history/condoms.shtml).

In the 1980s, the appearance of HIV and AIDS on the sexual playing field once again precipitated an increase in the use of condoms, although I think people stopped having sex altogether during the 1980s. Or maybe it was just us Generation Xers who were scared away from sex through the constant barrage of terrifying images of AIDS victims and the threat of HIV transmission. Fear as social control still works. Still, by the 1990s condom use was in full swing. In fact, the 1990s may even eventually be referred to as the golden age of the condom, the roaring nineties. Condom production in the 1990s exploded with the introduction of a large number of different styles, including various colored, ribbed, studded, and even flavored condoms. Moreover, the first polyurethane condom, catering to those allergic to latex, rolled out during the '90s. And now, in the new millennium, condoms are available in a wide array of sizes and shapes, thus rendering the problem of ill-fitting condoms obsolete. Indeed, although condoms have been around almost as long as the penis itself, custom-fitted condoms represent the latest evolutionary trend in condom manufacturing. Thankfully, people around the world no longer have to live in fear of accidentally inhaling a poorly fitted condom. Thank you, *Condomania*!

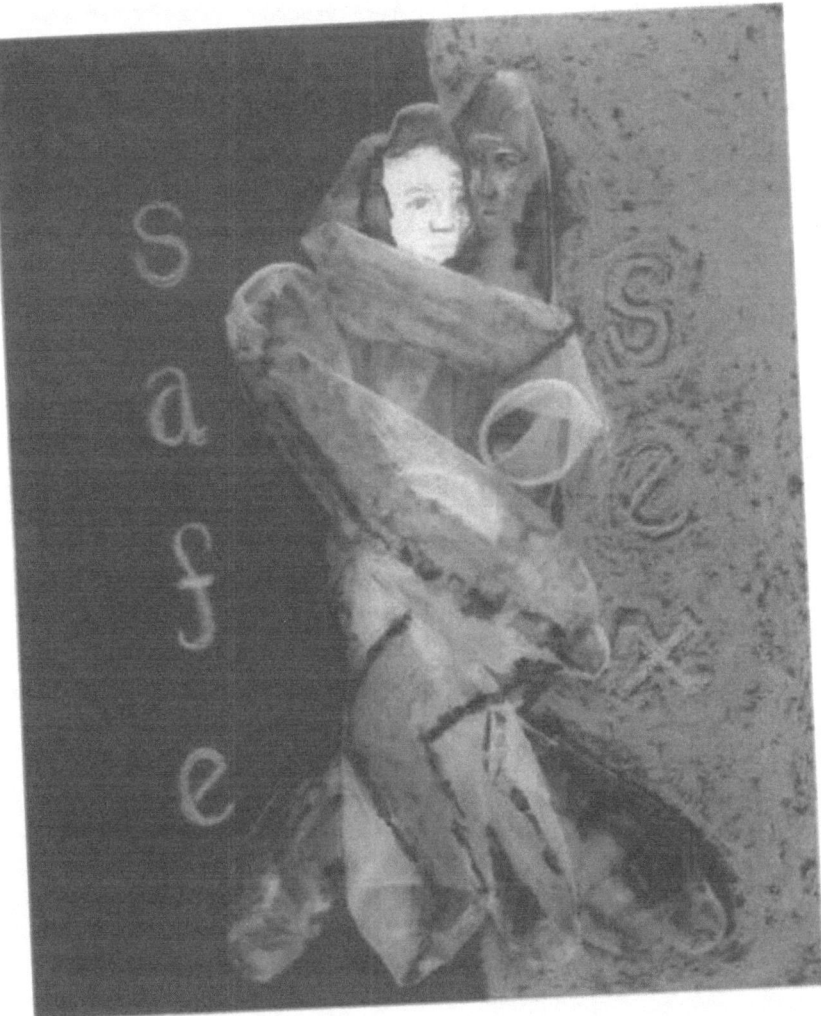

Safe Sex by Dominic Fetherston.

Notes

[1] Well, in 1950, of course. Who knows what the average penis length is for the same demographic now, given the number of "natural" human penis enlargement remedies currently available through e-mail SPAM and late night infomercials, but I'll get to those later!

[2] Internet site: *www.edu.uni-klu.ac.at/~amiklaut/dr_nick/answer19.htm.*

[3] This is keeping in line with the old adage, "When you assume, you make an ass out of you and me." Well, I may very well be an ass, but I've chosen to be conservative for ease of calculation.

[4] As opposed to Nanna-ometers, very large units of measurement!

[5] There are some different sizes available, but these "novelty" sizes usually cater to the over-endowed gentleman. As the name implies, a uniform distribution is one in which all values are equal.

[6] Some would argue that they already do, of course.

Bibliography

Arya, C. L., Gupta, R., & Arora, V. K. (2004). Accidental Condom Inhalation. *Indian Journal of Chest Diseases and Allied Sciences, 46*(1): 55–58.

Getzlaff, J. A. (2000). Germans too small for condoms? Available from: *www.salon.com/travel/planet/2000/03/06/condoms*

Herrnstein, R., and Murray, C. (1994). *The bell curve: Intelligence and class structure in American life.* New York: Simon and Schuster.

Internet site: *www.the-penis-website.com/condom.html.*

Internet site: *www.edu.uni-klu.ac.at/~amiklaut/dr_nick/answer19.htm.*

Internet site: *www.free-condom-stuff.com/fcs/html/penis-average-size.html.*

Internet site: *www.condomania.com.*

Internet site: *www.lifestyles.com/history/condoms.shtml.*

• CHAPTER EIGHT •

The Condom in History: Shame and Fear

Mark Lipton

Horses and latex gloves. In 1991, I was a part of the chorus of activists chanting "Money for AIDS, Not War!" just outside of Grand Central Terminal in New York City. As the crowd turned the corner, we saw the riot police marching on horseback toward us, about a block away. Word spread fast, something wasn't right, people were getting arrested. Weeks earlier, I had participated in one of ACT UP's civil disobedience training workshops, so I was prepared. As an activist, a member of this group, I knew what to do. No fear. But as a man in a crowd on the New York street, walking toward rows of cops on horseback, I admit I felt a little intimidated by the sounds of marching hooves. My first fear was of cops beating demonstrators bloody. It had happened before. "Shame" was the chant the crowd repeated as we walked past the cavalcade. Shame was being passed around like a ball. Shame on the city, the insurance companies, the drug companies. Shame on them for letting so many of us die. "Shame," I chanted as I pointed to the police. I was horrified. All the cops were wearing latex gloves. Why? Did they expect civil disobedience? A clash with the crowd to the point of violence? Did they expect blood? Were they afraid? The horses protected the police from the crowd; protection from AIDS took the form of latex. "Shame!" I shouted, shame on the police for not knowing better. I was afraid of what could happen next.

For the cops, the latex gloves served little purpose save for dishpan hands. But the gloves did provide a nervous law enforcement agency with something tangible to help quell the rising homophobia and AIDS-phobia among the force. Latex gloves were the answer because they provided a symbolic barrier between the world of AIDS and the world of the cops. There's nothing shameful about work in law enforcement. Shame is cast on homosexuals, the gay men and lesbians who don't live by God's law. Shame is cast on people with AIDS. In this context, shame is inexorably tied up with notions of fear. The best example is fear of contagion. The cops wanted to be protected from AIDS. To defend themselves against the AIDS enemy, the cops needed a protective strategy. To feel safe they turned to latex. Latex is the most obvious answer, because today's latex condoms are undoubtedly the most important means of contraception and, perhaps more significant, the most important means of preventing sexually transmitted infections (STIs).

There is a real stigma attached to all STIs. The changing language, from venereal diseases to sexually transmitted diseases to the name STI, signifies our culture's attempt to transcend the stigma associated with the language. But efforts to soften the stigma are not new. The use of condoms has been stressed historically for the prevention of syphilis and unwanted pregnancy. The shame of disease and fear of subsequent death as well as the shame of an unwanted birth and fear of its implications are vividly illustrated by the history of the condom. As will be demonstrated, condoms are the tool to prevent stigma. Condoms are part of the rich cultural history of shame and fear that account, in part, for many transformations among sexual affiliations and social ethics. A noted authority on the history of contraception, Dr. Norman E. Himes (1970), anticipated the social and cultural effects of the condom. "The vulcanization of rubber revolutionized transportation. Will it revolutionize morals and sexual relations? Time will give the safest verdict; but the answer seems clearly in the affirmative" (p. 186). To Himes, condoms are a medium of communication. He understands the ecology of media, how the evolution of this technology can have an effect on cultural values and beliefs. Himes believes that a culture of condoms will alter morals and sexual relations. A media ecological approach to studying an artifact's history attempts to understand its functions as well as purposes. The purpose of the condom certainly is to prevent unwanted pregnancies and the spread of STIs. Condoms are protection; their use involves a protective strategy. The functions of the condom consider the question of sexual relations and morality, that is, the social and cultural implications. There are other treatises on the history of the condom. The intention here is to take a media ecological position and examine the cultural importance of the condom's history.

A tablet from the Egyptian XII dynasty (1350–1200 B.C.) depicts a protective sheath covering the penis (Robertson, 1989, p. 112). These "penis protectors" were to act as shields against tropical diseases like *condirus* and *bilharzia* and against insect bites (Himes, 1970, p. 186). Though the actual material is unknown, they were probably made of clay or at least some "non-skin-like" material, signifying their function as other than the prevention of conception. These were a people clearly unconcerned with problems of population explosion or perfidious sexual relations. Egyptians were a people believed to use ritual to regulate such issues. Himes describes these "penis protectors" as serving some function of ritual; he suggests that condoms were used as badges of rank or status, amulets to promote fertility, or for decoration. These ritualistic possibilities cannot be completely confirmed, however, due to lack of surviving documentation. But right from its beginnings, the condom functioned as a protective strategy against a fear of tropical diseases.

Surprising to some, questions have been asked about condom use in imperial Rome. Much to the chagrin of traditional classicists, some interpretations of the mythology consider the condom as a protective strategy. This controversy is found in the legend of Minos and Pasiphaë. In the popular legend, Minos is remembered as not sacrificing a bull sent to him from Poseidon, the god of the sea. Poseidon then took his vengeance, inflicting Pasiphaë with an irresistible passion for the bull, and after much wooing, she conceived the monstrous Minotaur (Grant & Hazel, 1973, p. 281; Hamilton, 1969, pp. 151–2).

The more interesting story however, is about Minos's sex life. Having eight children, he and Pasiphaë were quite prolific. He also had five illegitimate children and mistresses so numerous that his envious wife was enraged. Possessing great skill as a sorceress, she put a curse on Minos so "all the women to whom he made love were devoured by serpents" (Grimal, 1991, p. 331). One modern interpretation of this consequence is that his lovers were afflicted by a sexually transmitted infection. The man with libidinous, carnal cravings is cursed by disease. The cultural attitude in this story suggests that sexually transmitted infections, disease, and death were adequate punishment for the morally wrong or abandoned. These feelings are echoed today, as judgment is wrongly placed on people afflicted by any kind of sexually transmitted infection.

Throughout the history of these infections, as discussed in the literature of venereology, there was always some form of treatment. At this point, the controversy of condom use enters. The goddess Procris, wanting Minos as a lover, supposedly supplied Minos with a cure. How she healed Minos, however, is in question. Some suggestions point directly to the invention of a proto-condom as means of treatment. Antoninus Liberalis's treatment of the myth illustrates this possibility: "She [Procris] slipped the bladder of a goat into the vagina of a woman. Into this bladder Minos cast off his serpent-bearing semen. Then he went to find Pasiphaë, and cohabited with her" (Liberalis, 1992, p. 142). Assuming this legend reflects the practices and customs of Imperial Rome, it can be said that the bladders of animals were used to receive the sperm of men during intercourse with the purpose of protecting women against the consequence of pregnancy or infection. Whatever the motivation, this story describes a culture that placed some value on monogamy, where disease is a consequence of promiscuity. For Procris, the condom is a protective strategy to deal with her fear of contracting Minos's ailment.

This story also illuminates gender relations and the concept of the body in imperial Rome. The prevention of disease was the woman's concern. It was Procris, and not a man, who devised the method of prevention, and consequently conceived it to be worn by a woman; it was a female sheath. The concern of prevention was gender-related; Roman women had to pay the price of caution when engaging in promiscuous practices. Men were seemingly ignorant. Pasiphaë "transmitted" the affliction, and Procris supplied the treatment. Minos was the impervious carrier, passing the disease to "all the women to whom he made love." The role of men is omitted in all interpretations of this myth, demonstrating the beginnings of a cultural record of gender-biased relations. By inventing the female condom, Procris put the responsibility of sex and its repercussions into the hands of women, giving men greater sexual freedom.

This power extends to the notion of sexual relations without women. Homosexuality is a viable application of the power granted to the masculine and clearly was ethically acceptable to the Romans. Pasiphaë's curse inflicted only other women. The fact that only women were at risk of infection privileges a narcissistic worship of the male body. It is not a coincidence that this issue comes up at this point in the story. Many scholars consider Minos as the originator of homosexuality. "In one tradition Minos rather than Zeus abducted Ganymede. He is also said to be the lover of Theseus and was supposedly reconciled with him after Ariadne's abduction, and gave him his daughter Phaedra in marriage" (Grimal, 1991, p. 276). Apparently Minos did not infect his male partners, further privileging the masculine. The stigma of homosexuality did not exist; rather, it was an acceptable form of behavior. Men could love other men freely, but loving women brought the responsibility of procreation. There is no analytic discussion or debate over the morality of homosexuality, and thus it is untenable to suggest that one form of sexual relations was preferred or more sacred. The approbation of homosexual relations, however, illustrates as a truism that sex for pleasure was not considered a deviant form of behavior in ancient Rome, and there were significant gender differences when dealing with the body. Oh, the arrogance of Minos.

The first official "published" description of the condom appears in 1564 when Gabrielle Fallopius's *De morbo gallico* describes a linen sheath serving as protection against syphilis. This sheath had to be fitted; it was cut to fit the tip of the penis and the foreskin was pulled over it. Fallopius, one of the early authorities, claims to have been its inventor. He describes the process (here reproduced in translation):

> As often as a man has intercourse, he should (if possible) wash the genitals, or wipe them with a cloth; afterward he should use a small linen cloth made to fit the glans, and draw forward the prepuce over the glans; if he can do so, it is well to moisten it with saliva or with a lotion; however, it does not matter: If you fear lest caries [syphilis] be produced [in] the canal, take the sheath of the linen cloth and place it in the canal; I tried the experiment on eleven hundred men, and I call immortal God to witness that not one of them was infected. (Himes, 1970, p. 190)

Fallopius's early condom was significantly different from the condoms of today. Like today's condoms, however, the linen sheath had the advantage of portability; this condom could be carried around in a pocket, which allowed sexual activity to occur at any time or place. Instantaneous sex was probably something not unknown, but now a man could greatly reduce the risk of infection by being prepared. Sex was now accompanied by a technology, but sexual freedom brought with it responsibility. Men had to think ahead, and cut (or have made) a condom to fit their glans. The penis now had an appendage for protection. This appendage allowed a shift to occur between what was considered right and wrong. What was right used to be an act of restraint, not engaging in sex. But now, with a condom, what was right was to engage in acts of protected sex.

Fallopius clearly put the power of sexual relations into the hands of men. His condom is a sheath produced for men, to be used by men. Men are offered the power and freedom to break existing sexual rules without suffering the consequences. Out of eleven hundred men, not one was infected with syphilis. It is important to stress here that the entire purpose of Fallopius's linen sheath was to protect men against infection. The stigma of sinfulness was imprinted on syphilis, and it was the fear of disease that shamed men into using the condom as a protective strategy. The only affiliation with women was to acknowledge them as the object of sex. Fallopius illustrates this power when he describes the process of putting the sheath into the vagina, if syphilis were suspected. How to determine whether or not a woman was infected was left up to the man's speculation.

This gender-biased distinction is furthered by Fallopius's avowal to "immortal God." The presence of God identifies the ethical politics surrounding Fallopius's condom. The condom as an appendage to sexual activity was apparently not unethical; immorality came with the infection of syphilis. Infection was a well-deserved punishment that visited offenders who broke ethical and natural laws. By calling "immortal God to witness," Fallopius's scientific study morally sanctions men's sexual freedom. It is not wrong for men to be promiscuous, as long as they do not get caught with their pants down.

After Fallopius's mention of the protective linen sheath, the information was passed down through an enormous amount of literature on syphilis. It is in this collection of work, around the seventeenth century, that the word "condom" is introduced. "Condum" is initially used by Daniel Turner, an English physician, in 1717. He describes its unpopularity:

> The *Condum* being the best, if not only Preservative our Libertines have found out at present; and yet by reason of its blunting the Sensation, I have heard some of them acknowledge, that they had often chose to risk a *Clap*, rather than engage *cum Hastis sic clypeatis* [with spears thus sheathed]. (Langley, 1973, p. 81)

By reporting the condom as uncomfortable, "blunting the sensation," Turner emphasizes the importance of sexual pleasure. Sensual gratification is dulled with Fallopius's appendage to sexual activity. According to Turner, condoms ridicule masculinity by stressing disease prevention over sensual pleasure. The ethical stance is clear; condoms are not a necessary part of sex, as Fallopius suggests, but an unnecessary and uncomfortable attachment.

Thus begins the cultural disdain of the condom. Though the sheath was in general use in Europe by 1671 (Robertson, 1989, p. 113), no one wants to claim credit for the introduction of the word. Neither the French nor the English care to accept initial recognition. The French place blame with their expression *la capote anglaise* (the English cape). The English reciprocate with the term "French letter," emphasizing the French origin (Robertson, 1989, p. 114).

Many theories have evolved to account for the possible etymology of the word. E. L. Bernstein (1940), for example, dedicated an article titled "Who Was Condom?" to the intricacies of the word's possible etymology. If from the French, condom could be similar to *condamne*, meaning a condemned person, or *condus*, a form of the verb *condere*, "that which preserves." If from the English, there is great debate about the possibility of Condom as a proper name. Bernstein articulates this argument, concluding, "*Cundum* did exist. He was an Englishman" (Bernstein in Langley, 1973, p. 85). Other theorists are not as certain. Havelock Ellis (1936), for example, discussed other possibilities.

> The name, "condom," dates from the eighteenth century, first appearing in France, and is generally considered to be that of an English physician, or surgeon, who invented, or, rather, improved the appliance. Condom is not, however, an English name, but there is an English name, Condon, of which "condom" may well be a corruption. (p. 600)

In the literature of venereology, it is most commonly stated that the condom was invented by, and named after, one Dr. Condon, a physician at the court of Charles II (Himes, 1970, p. 192; Bernstein in Langley, 1973, p. 174; Robertson, 1989, p. 113). This too is heavily debated. Ellis (1936) explained the difficulty of discovering any Englishman named Condon who can plausibly be associated with the instrument: "Doubtless he took no care to put the matter on record, never suspecting the fame that would accrue to his invention, or the immortality that awaited his name" (p. 600).

The connection between the condom and Charles II is of particular interest. Apparently the king did not like having so many illegitimate children. Eric Delderfield (1988) acknowledges King Charles's thirteen known mistresses. Of twenty-six dukes living in England today, five are direct descendants of Charles II (p. 88). Certainly the king would be annoyed by his misbegotten children, but these children may have also disturbed the church. In examining the history of the Church of England, Charles II is associated with the beginnings of religious toleration. Henry Wakeman (1908) describes Charles's attitude: "He [Charles] turned for support during the rest of his reign to the militant Churchmen, and in return for their doctrine of passive obedience cynically surrendered the nonconformists to the operation of the penal laws" (p. 395). Bishop Henry *Compton* of London was one such "Churchman," and though this may be a stretch, it is possible that the bishop gave Charles an instrument (a "Compton" or a "condom") to appease the Church. If you account for regional dialects and printing techniques, this may not be any more of a corruption than "condon." (The mind soars.)

Though this possibility may explain some of the contradictory theories, the implications are enormous, especially for the Church and the religious conflicts of the time. But it is only a theory and like the other theories, I am inclined to think it a myth and confess that proof is impossible, but disproof too is impossible in light of all the debate. The real inventor probably hit upon the idea by accident, is unknown, and never will be known. The name aside, at this point in its history, the condom helped give birth to new worldviews about sex, to varying ethical points of view about disease, and to some differences between the sexes. In short, condoms function as the best protective strategy against fear and shame. The fact that no one has staked a claim to the name reinforces the stigma of unwanted pregnancy or infection.

Jacques Casanova de Seingalt had no problem with using a condom. He used natural skin condoms in the middle of the eighteenth century, referring to them as "English riding coats, which puts one's mind at rest" (Himes, 1970, p. 195). Casanova used condoms not only to prevent infection, but to avoid impregnating his women. According to his memoirs, on All Saints' Day in 1753, he used condoms when engaging in sex with a Viennese nun. On another occasion, about to enter into relations with a "public" woman, he admitted to her his fear of possible infection. In response, she produced a box of condoms that mollified Casanova's fears (Himes, 1970, p. 195). Casanova is candid about his sexual endeavors, symbolizing a new approach to sex. By the end of the eighteenth century, sexual freedom comes with a social and ethical responsibility. Casanova demonstrates through his use of the condom how men must show care to avoid disease or unwanted pregnancy. What he puts on his body is a significant tool prohibiting an exchange of bodily fluids.

Though Casanova's open attitude is an exception in many ways, gender distinctions continue to be illustrated in his account. Although women are portrayed as sexual, from nun to prostitute, they are still treated as the objects of male sexual pleasure. The Viennese nun in Casanova's story demonstrates how men must protect themselves from social and ethical harm. To impregnate a nun would represent a violation of religious virtue. The "public" woman, on the other hand, might infect Casanova with an illness, leaving him unable to continue with his sexual antics. Women are always the cause of some problem to which the condom is the solution.

It is important to note that Casanova's exceptional story does not reflect the general feeling about condoms. In the literature of venereology, condoms are discussed with disdain. In 1738 Johannes Astruc, for one, describes condom use in his treatise on venereal disease.

> I hear from the lowest debauchees who chase without restraint after the love of prostitutes, that there are recently employed in England skins made from soft and seamless hides in the shape of a sheath, and called condoms in English, with which those about to have intercourse wrap their penis as in a coat of mail in order to render themselves safe in the dangers of an ever doubtful battle. They claim, I

suppose, that thus mailed and with spears sheathed in this way, they can undergo with impunity the chances of promiscuous intercourse. But (in truth) they are greatly mistaken. (Himes, 1970, p. 196)

What "they are greatly mistaken" about, according to Astruc, is within the arena of ethics and morality. His description of men as "the lowest debauchees who chase without restraint" clearly signifies condom users as lacking ethics; these men are corrupt and perverted. The condom, for Astruc, is the signifier of evil and sin. These men should be ashamed. Condoms emerge as the technology that measure a man's level of morality. The more one chases "without restraint," the more debauched, the lower the morality.

Nonetheless, the sale of condoms eventually became a part of business; condoms were sold openly and vigorously in the latter part of the eighteenth century. In 1776, a Mrs. Philips of Half Moon Street in London distributed handbills advertising the sale of condoms of high quality at her establishment, the Green Cannister. These handbills describe her goods and who buys them, and they affirm her business as authentic. They read:

To guard yourself from shame and fear,
Votaries to Venus, hasten here;
None in my wares e'er found a flaw,
Self preservation's nature's law.

By describing condoms as a guard against shame and fear, Mrs. Philips describes the purposes as protective strategies, against an unwanted pregnancy (shame) and against disease (fear). Though these two purposes are often separated, looked at through different lenses and thought of as having different consequences, Mrs. Philips introduces the notion of protection as the key element. Self-preservation is nature's law. Her standpoint is neither religious nor perverted; all must guard themselves from shame and fear. Again it is important to note that the clientele to whom Mrs. Phillips sells her wares are men. At least publicly, it is men who must guard themselves, and it is *themselves* they must guard, not their female sexual partners.

Widespread, common use of the condom had to await the vulcanization of rubber. First carried out by Goodyear in 1843, this process so significantly lowered the cost of production that every nineteenth- and twentieth-century treatise dealing with sexual technique gave condoms a prominent place (Himes, 1970, p. 201). Condoms achieved even greater access by the use of liquid latex and automatic machinery, introduced in the early 1930s. Today, latex condoms are the primary technique employed for the prevention of the unwanted infection and pregnancy. Since latex condoms are the only sufficient barrier against HIV disease, they are the only sexual strategy to prevent both the shame and fear of AIDS.

There are many people who still find condom use problematic. Condoms are either too uncomfortable, frustrate spontaneity, or dull the sensation for men. As a result, it should be of little surprise that the close of the twentieth century saw the production and distribution of the "female condom." The Wisconsin Pharmacal company was granted federal approval of Reality, the "intravaginal pouch." This product claims to put the power of control into the hands of women. But, like the proto-condom of Procris, Reality is divorced from any sexual revolution and returns men to that point in history where women took up the concern of protection. Let us not forget that the proto-condom of Procris reinforced gender-biased relations, privileging men. Because of cost, awkwardness of use, and limited availability, the female condom is amusement at best. It is another attempt to provide our culture with a protective strategy against shame and fear.

In the age of AIDS, what can and cannot be put into the body has become especially important to members of Western culture. Fear of AIDS and its subsequent stigma has invigorated a culture of condoms. As information on the transmission of HIV disseminates into public knowledge, the exchange of bodily fluids is feared, as it may lead to some form of shame or shameful death. It is not coincidence that with the drastic fear of AIDS comes a caution of what is put into the body, the fear of bodily fluids. We all must show care when allowing something to enter our bodies, and condoms are the leading tool controlling the gates. The "Health" crusade can be thought of as an extension of condom culture. We are all concerned to prevent unwanted substances from entering our bodies, whether they are semen, blood, or cholesterol. Of course, it isn't that simple. And using condoms isn't that easy either. Just look to the rising numbers of young gay men who openly engage in unsafe sex, a practice called "barebacking." Why are young people today not using condoms? Why are condoms so stigmatized in other parts of the world? Again, part of the answer is about shame and fear. In the twenty-first century, there is no shame in homosexuality. There is no shame in contracting HIV disease. In the age of highly active anti-retroviral therapy, the venerable AIDS cocktails, there is no point to fear, no time for fear. It seems easy to deny the culture of condoms. AIDS apartheid divides the gay community, negative men on one side, afraid of their positive counterparts. No point to shame, too late for shame. So with or without the condom, it is undeniable that today we live in a latex culture. By discussing the history of the condom, I hope to provide a platform or a departure point from which to learn about effective protective strategies in the fight against STIs. The best way to initiate communication about sex with young people is to bring up the subject of condoms. Safer sex is part of our cultural landscape, and young people are savvy to the culture of condoms.

In conclusion, condoms have played a hand in developing Western cultural norms, values, and attitudes. Condoms have allowed people to overcome fear: a fear of disease, a fear of death, a fear of shame; and in the process, condoms have altered what is right and wrong. As we continue to live in the age of AIDS, condoms will continue to contribute to our social atmosphere and cultural climate. We are all people living with AIDS, and until there is a cure, we are also a people living and loving with condoms.

Bibliography

Abbey, C. (1887). *The English church and its bishops.* London: Longmans, Green, and Co.

Delderfield, E. A. (1988). *Kings and queens of England.* Dorset Press: New York.

De Seingalt, J. C. (translated by Machen, A.). (1932). *The memories of Jacques Casanova de Seingalt, Volumes I, II, & III.* New York: Dover Publications Inc.

Ellis, H. (1936). *Studies in the psychology of sex, Volume IV.* New York: Random House.

Fallopius, G. (1564). *De morbo gallico.*

Grant, M., and Hazel, J. (1973). *Gods and mortals in classical mythology.* Stroudsburg, PA: Dowden, Hutchinson & Ross, Inc.

Grimal, P. (1991). *Dictionary of classical mythology.* New York: Penguin.

Hamilton, E. (1969). *Mythology: Timeless tales of gods and heroes.* Scarborough, Ontario: Mentor.

———. (1980). *The illustrious lady*. London: Hamish Hamilton.

Himes, N. E. (1970). *Medical history of contraception*. New York: Schocken Books.

Langley, L. L. (Ed.). (1973). *Contraception*. Springfield, MA: G&C Merriam Company.

Liberalis, A. (1992). *The metamorphoses of Antoninus Liberalis*. Francis Celoria (trans.) London and New York: Routledge.

Pearson, H. (1960). *Charles II: His life and likeness*. Toronto: Heinemann.

Robertson, W. H. (1989). *An illustrated history of contraception*. New Jersey: The Parthenon Publishing Group.

Stokes, J. (1919). Today's world problem in disease prevention. Washington, D.C.: U.S. Public Health Service.

Turner, D. (1717). *A practical treatise on the venereal disease*. London.

Wakeman, H. O. (1908). *An introduction to the history of the church of England*. London: Rivingtons.

• CHAPTER NINE •

Stiff Competition:
A Thrust for Condom Education

Devon C. Adams

Planned Parenthood of Western Pennsylvania's Action Fund (PPWPAF) has engaged in a creative approach to promote condom education. The committee originated the idea of a condom art competition in the summer of 1992, upon identifying an untapped young artist population in Pittsburgh likely to be pro-choice and liberal. During the premiere year of the event (now known as the Stiff Competition), the Action Fund issued a slick call for entries, which generated a list of artists and designers in the tri-state area of Western Pennsylvania, Eastern Ohio, and West Virginia.

The committee asked for a wrapper design that would capture a Pittsburgh theme, searching for the "quintessential Pittsburgh condom packaging." Thirty designers accepted the challenge the first year, while four years later the entry number rose to over one hundred, and the finalists' works were displayed at the Andy Warhol Museum on Pittsburgh's North Side during the month of June. In 2004, the panel of judges included Mattress Factory Director Barbara Luderowski, Three Rivers Arts Festival Director Elizabeth Reiss, Concept Art gallery owner Sam Berkovitz, Mendelson Gallery owner Steven Mendelson, and Pittsburgh Public Theater Artistic Director Ted Pappas. They chose a first, second, and third place design, in addition to several comical ad hoc categories.

The event continues to grow and expand. Over three hundred people attended last year's art auction, where the winning designs were sold and reproduced on condom packaging. They are sold online at www.stiffcompetition.org. Last year's winners included "Some Like It On," a parody of the film *Some Like It Hot*, featuring Marilyn Monroe's lascivious lips with the tag line, "Some Like It On. Coming Soon...to the bedrooms near you."

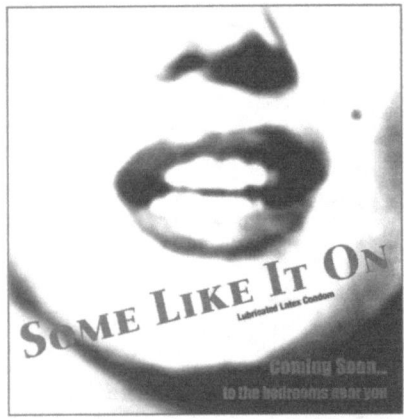

Second place was awarded to an ad entitled "Greased," featuring an artistic rendition similar to the movie poster for the film *Grease,* although this representation includes a pair of feminine legs jutting askew from the rear seat of the vehicle.

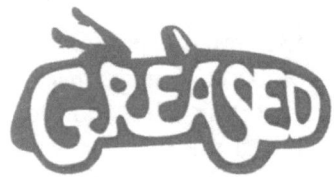

LUBRICATED CONDOMS

Third place parodied the 1970s blaxploitation film *Shaft,* with a man asking his partner if he or she can "dig it?"

Each year the Action Fund chooses themes based on political and cultural references to current situations in the region and in our country.

Reflecting and responding to current political, social, and cultural exigencies in the region, indeed, in the whole country, the Action Fund's themes have included "Stiff Competition: Where Safe Sex Meets Pop Art," which encouraged designers to mesh pop art with the culture of the city; "Stiff Competition II: The Second Coming: A Landmark Decision," which asked the artists to design the quintessential condom based on famous Pittsburgh landmarks; and "Stiff Competition III: A Hard Look at Local History," designed to showcase famous, or infamous, Pittsburgh history. The fourth competition was entitled "Hollywood: A Hard Act to Follow," while the 2004 contest is "Presidential Condoms: When Politics Makes for Strange Bedfellows."

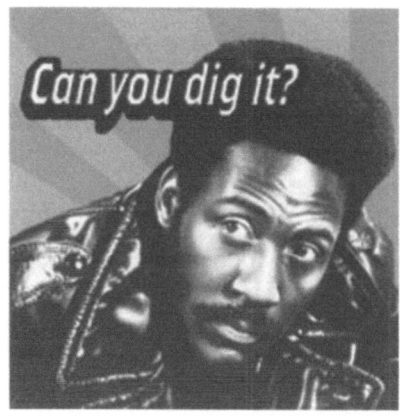

While the Stiff Competition was established locally to publicize safe sex and condom use in a regional way, due to its continued publicity and popularity, coupled with an appeal to a diverse market, the competition expanded globally and gained momentum as it moved from word of mouth to the Internet.

Initially the event made $14,000; this figure has increased to $16,500, even though significant expenditures are involved. Many of the supporters of Stiff Competition remain unaware that they are supporting Planned Parenthood as the parent group of the competition. Jodi Hirsh, director of public affairs, found it disconcerting that Planned Parenthood's involvement is practically invisible in this contest, as the excitement of the contest, themes, and gala itself take precedence.

The thrust of the Stiff Competition is to globally educate on the message of safe sex, condom use, and the need to become politically and civically involved in a creative way, while Planned Parenthood of Western Pennsylvania's Action Fund engages in educational and political issues including issues in education, grassroots organizing, public opinion research, lobbying, and independent expenditure campaigns.

Bibliography

Stiff Competition 2004. *Presidential Condoms: When Politics Makes for Strange Bedfellows*. Planned Parenthood of Western Pennsylvania Action Fund.

• CHAPTER TEN •

Engineering the Condom

Charla Triplett

Most people rarely think about how products are made. We might hear about the latest engineering advance in a car or cell phone commercial, but how often do we contemplate how side airbags or cameras in our phones affect our lives? Engineers design and manufacture just about every consumer product imaginable, including condoms. Though we may not consciously realize it, this engineering influence is felt in most aspects of our lives, even our reproductive health. Marxist theory assumes that products become a reflection of the laborers themselves. If this is true, then clearly the white heterosexual male is reflected in the condom, since engineers are still overwhelmingly a homogenous population. The condom is a unique product, because it is intrinsically wrapped up with sexuality and gender roles. Who chooses the method of contraception, who buys it, and how it is ultimately used are issues that are intertwined with sexual freedom and power.

Engineering as a field is relatively uninterested in such ideas; it is all about innovation and design. Engineers are not trained, in general, to contemplate the ethical, moral, or political implications of their work. The focus is on product improvement and scientific progress. As Linda Shepherd (1993) states in her book *Lifting the Veil: The Feminine Face of Science*, "Science seems to promote a technological imperative like manifest destiny. We rarely consider the values built into new technology or how applications of science change the social patterns and daily lives of people" (p. 109).

Engineers may have the capacity to create novel technologies, but profit drives what actually makes it to the market. Think about how many "advances" have been made in the toothbrush or the disposable razor in the past few years. It seems every week competitors come out with new bells and whistles. Unfortunately for the condom, the advertising and marketing that drives all those new features is not widely available. The only place you are likely to see a condom ad is on MTV, in an adult magazine, or, more recently, the Internet. Cyberspace has opened up new ground for condom advertising with condom banner ads. New marketing campaigns also target college students with spring break freebies and a Trojan brand condom screen saver (Digital Perks web site). Perhaps these new approaches will allow companies to pursue specialized condom production more effectively.

In addition to advertising limitations, the condom is a special type of product categorized as a medical device, which means that any significant changes in the design must go through the Food and Drug Administration (FDA) regulatory process like any other medical device, such as a pacemaker or artificial hip (FDA Medical Device web site). While regulation and advertising may limit the dollars that are put into condom innovation, actual consumer preferences may be masked by the embarrassment of standing in the condom aisle trying to decide which brand has the better features. These factors perhaps point to the reason why the condom has not quite kept up with other drugstore products in "advancing technology."

Condoms have been around for centuries, but the modern latex version that we are most familiar with was not widely used until the 1930s. The basic design requirements of the condom are that it must be shaped to provide adequate covering, remain tight enough to stay on during intercourse (yet expand to accommodate a range of lengths and widths), maintain its strength and integrity during intercourse, and be made of a material that is compatible with the body but does not allow sperm to escape its pores. Early condoms were made from animal membranes and intestines, and even linen. They were often no more than crude wrappings. The invention of vulcanized rubber created the ability to mass-produce condoms in the mid-1800s, and thus the term "rubber" was coined. Eventually, latex became the ultimate material of choice because of its cost and reliability compared with other materials.

Unfortunately, the one time engineering does make the news is when there is a design flaw or failure. We can all identify with the impact of a space shuttle disaster or a bridge that collapses, but very few inexpensive products can have the kind of long-term individual consequences that condom failure can. Even when used properly, condoms have a 2 percent failure rate, which means that two out of every one hundred condoms will break or leak. The actual failure rate is closer to 10 percent due to improper use, because the best design and testing cannot prevent user error or carelessness (Global Protection Corporation web site). This fact has long been used as an excuse to have women bear the responsibility of birth control, since the Pill has a lower rate of failure. The availability of the morning-after pill, in conjunction with condom use, now makes this argument obsolete and affords women a greater level of control over unplanned pregnancy, disease prevention, and hormone usage.

The advent of AIDS in the 1980s increased condom usage when research studies demonstrated that they provided protection against HIV in addition to pregnancy. The sexual revolution brought about by the Pill was not without health risks. While the long-term consequences of sexual choices have always been an issue for women, now men too must consider the life-altering effects of sex. As Rosalind Coward (1996) puts it in her chapter from *Feminism and Sexuality*, "The Pill allowed women an unprecedented degree of spontaneity, but it could hardly be described as unpremeditated or unrisky...but now, suddenly it's a matter of life and death to men that they abandon their historical privilege of spontaneous sex and assume personal responsibility for their actions" (p. 246).

Currently about 13 billion condoms are manufactured worldwide annually. Over 600 million are sold each year in the United States alone, a large number of condoms that make it from the manufacturing plant into consumers' hands. In order to ensure reliability, every condom is put through individual electronic testing, which consists of the condom being stretched over metal and exposed to an electrical field. Because the condom should not conduct electricity, the field should not reach the metal. If it does, that indicates pinholes and the condom will be discarded (Global Protection Corporation web site).

In addition to this individual testing, condoms from each lot are randomly tested. In the dimensions test, the length, width, and thickness of the condoms are measured, and if a certain number of condoms are out of acceptable range, the lot is rejected. During the tensile properties test, a ring is cut from the condom and then stretched until breakage. The force required to break the condom is measured and recorded for quality control. Condoms are hung vertically and filled with water during the leakage test, and for the air burst test, they are blown up like balloons. Finally, package testing makes sure that the condoms are sealed correctly. Statistics are used to analyze these tests, and lots that fall below the acceptable failure range are discarded. This allows for increased reliability without the need to perform each of these tests on every condom manufactured (Global Protection Corporation web site).

Though improvements have been slow in the past, the last decade has brought several new condom innovations. A look at the advances in condom design will show, for example, the invention of the reservoir tip, which allows for rubbing back and forth during intercourse, said to enhance pleasure for both partners. In addition to the traditional ribbed condom, there are new versions specifically designed for female sensation, with ribs at the base of the condom. Another new popular design, the Inspiral, twists up like a double helix when put on and creates friction when used. Intellx, the company that manufactures the Inspiral, is using manufacturing techniques that allow for unique asymmetrical shapes, not considered possible in mass production ten years ago (Intellx Inc. web site).

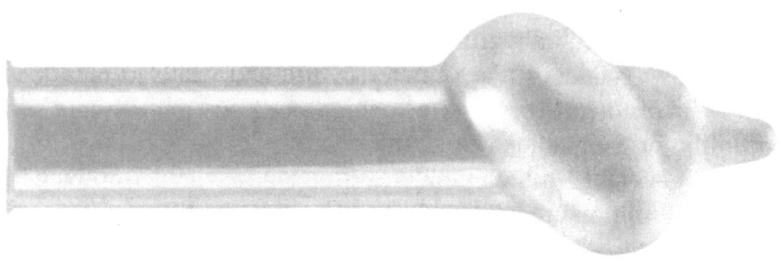

Image of Inspiral Condom, Intellx Inc.

Flavored condoms have been around for a while, but until recently those were more novelty items than for actual protective use. Several new lines of flavored condoms have now been approved by the FDA, with flavors like banana, grape, vanilla, chocolate, and cola. High-quality glow-in-the-dark condoms are also now available, intended for the prevention of pregnancy and disease as well as entertainment. Finally, for those with premature ejaculation problems, a line of condoms with the numbing agent benzocaine has been introduced.

The approval of polyurethane for use as a condom material created an acceptable substitute for latex. While lambskin condoms were an option for those with a latex allergy, the material had pore sizes that allowed some viruses to get through and did not provide adequate disease protection. Another benefit is that polyurethane does not weaken like latex with the use of oil-based lubricants. Water-based lubricants and spermicides are currently the only options for use with latex. Nonoxynol-9, the most common spermicide added to condoms, was once thought to help prevent HIV infections. However, more recent studies have shown that irritation caused by the substance may actually increase the transmission of certain sexually transmitted diseases.

Probably the greatest condom innovation in the last decade was the introduction of the female condom. Not only is this condom made of a new material, polyurethane, but it also has other features that make it possibly does not need to be removed immediately after ejaculation. The female condom also has social implications. It is being distributed in many countries to sex workers and other women who have little say in asking partners to use male condoms.

The use of the female condom can empower women and increase the protection against unwanted pregnancy and sexually transmitted diseases. It is notable that the company that designed the first female condom has a female president, and the design team was led by female engineers. With women still greatly underrepresented in the engineering field, perhaps that is what it took to create the female condom. The company also works closely with the Female Health Foundation, a nonprofit organization dedicated to improving sexual, reproductive, and family health by elevating awareness of women's health issues throughout the world. The first latex female condom, shown below, is currently being distributed in Europe, and should soon be available in the United States (Intellx Inc. web site).

Condoms have become commonplace during the past twenty years, and their role in our culture has changed, as they have gone from primarily birth control devices to potentially life-saving devices. Marketing phrases like "ribbed for her pleasure" make it clear that the condom manufacturers are considering both men and women in their design. Though the traditional condom is worn by men, both men and women use the product during heterosexual intercourse. A UK study in the nineties showed that 80 percent of women and 70 percent of men used condoms during their first sexual experience (Segal, 1997). These numbers are more than double that of previous decades. As Marla Singer, the self-help junkie from *Fight Club*, put it, "The condom is the glass slipper of our generation. You slip it on when you meet a stranger, dance all night, and then throw it away. The condom, I mean, not the stranger."

With advances in biomaterials, the future of the condom looks bright. High-tech patents have been filed for a condom with a self-stiffening agent that gets hard with the motion of sexual intercourse and a condom lined with a transdermal patch to release a chemical agent that enhances an erection (Levins, 1996). Soon there may be an "invisible condom," which is actually a gel, liquid at room temperature, that solidifies to coat the vagina at body temperature. It is currently being tested, and if it proves effective, could offer a novel addition to the realm of condoms.

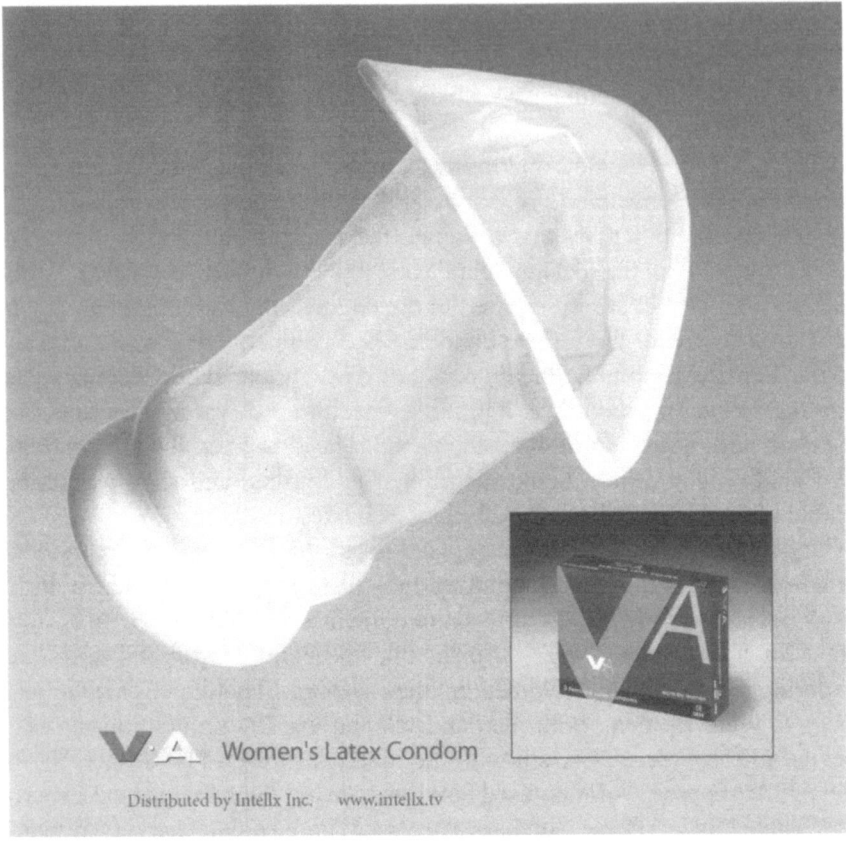

In addition to these inventions, Lifestyles has introduced a new foil-top condom package that resembles an individually wrapped pat of butter. It has easy-open tabs that peel back to reveal a condom that is right side up; maybe not quite as exciting as other advancements, but it certainly could solve one of the major complaints of condom users.

Other companies are looking at condom designs better suited for gay men. With advances in science and engineering, condoms have come a long way from the days when they were made from animal intestines. As the future of engineering changes, perhaps we will see the male condom change fundamentally as well. Biomedical engineering students nationwide are almost 50 percent female; surely their influence will be felt in the contraceptive products of the next generation.

Bibliography

Condomania web site: *www.condomania.com.*

Coward, R. (1996). Sex after AIDS. In S. Jackson and S. Scott (Eds.), *Feminism and sexuality: Gender and culture reader.* Edinburgh: Edinburgh University Press.

Digital Perks web site: *www.digitalperks.com/pitchitbanners.phtml.*

FDA Medical Device web site: *www.fda.gov/cdrh/index.html.*

Female Health Corporation web site: *www.femalehealth.com.*

Global Protection Corporation web site: *www.globalprotection.com.*

Intellx Inc. web site: *http://inspiral.tv.*

Levins, H. (1996). *American sex machines: The hidden history of sex at the patent office.* Avon, MA: Adams Media Publications.

McNeill, E., Gilmore, C., Finger, R., Lewis, J., and Schellstede, W. (1998). *The latex condom: Recent advances, future directions.* Research Triangle Park, NC: Family Health International.

Segal, L. (1997). Sexual liberation and feminist politics. In S. Kemp and J. Squires (Eds.), *Feminisms.* Oxford, UK: Oxford University Press.

Shepherd, L. J. (1993). *Lifting the veil: The feminine face of science.* Boston: Shambhala Publications, Inc.

• CHAPTER ELEVEN •

Sanctioned Discourse: Women, Condoms, and HIV/AIDS in Early 1990s Government Brochures

Dacia Charlesworth

By the end of 2003, the World Health Organization reported that 19.2 million women were living with human immunodeficiency virus/acquired immunodeficiency virus (HIV/AIDS) worldwide and accounted for 50 percent of the 40 million adults living with HIV/AIDS (National Institute of Allergy and Infectious Diseases, 2004). In the United States, the Centers for Disease Control (CDC, 2000a) report that HIV infection in women has increased significantly during the last decade. The CDC also note that although African-American and Hispanic women account for less than one-fourth of the population of U.S. women, they account for more than three-fourths of AIDS cases among U. S. women. In fact, AIDS remains the leading cause of death among African-American women aged 25–44 (CDC, 2000b).

Although no one would doubt that women are currently affected by HIV/AIDS, women's risk of becoming infected with HIV was not recognized until the early 1990s. In fact, it took the government until 1993 before the National Institute of Allergy and Infectious Diseases conducted a large-scale study to investigate the impact of HIV on women in the United States (CDC, 1993b). In that same year, the Food and Drug Administration (FDA) finally changed a 1977 policy that excluded most women capable of becoming pregnant from important clinical trials and also issued a guideline to encourage pharmaceutical companies to include women in reasonable numbers and to report any significant differences between women and men in their responses in drug trials to the FDA (Willis, 1997). Thus, women's identities in the HIV/AIDS pandemic (i.e., as individuals at risk of becoming infected with HIV) began to be formed by governmental agencies in the early 1990s.

The purpose of this essay, then, is to examine the sanctioned discourse of safe sex, especially as it relates to condom use, generated by governmental agencies and targeted to women when their "at risk" status was first identified in the early 1990s. To determine how these identities were developed, I examine one form of discourse generated for mass consumption: HIV/AIDS public education brochures. These brochures offer a particularly useful site for exploring the cultural, rhetorical, and ideological dimensions used to construct public identities in the AIDS pandemic. For example, they can be directed to a very general audience or a very specific audience, are relatively inexpensive to produce, and have the potential to reach large populations. My findings suggest that through these brochures the government places women of color in a double bind, because although they acknowledge women of color as being "at risk," they address these women by reifying cultural and class distinctions that ultimately serve to stigmatize them. In addition, the government does a disservice to its citizens by communicating about condom usage in a vague manner that seems more intent on not offending readers than educating them. I begin by discussing the method of analysis for the present study. Next, I offer an analysis of AIDS brochures directed at women. Finally, I draw conclusions as to the impact of these messages for women and men almost ten years later.

Methodology

I utilized a volunteer sample to collect the 40 brochures analyzed in this study. A form letter was mailed to national, state, and local health organizations soliciting any and all educational brochures they had pertaining to women and HIV/AIDS. It is significant that these agencies also included brochures targeted to other populations (e.g., gay men and IV drug users) along with information about women. Although those brochures are not targeted specifically to women, they do contain information about women's identities and serve as another valuable site to discover how women's identities are constructed for other audiences; thus, I have included them in my sample. In addition, I am also including brochures from private organizations so that I may compare their messages about condom usage to the messages prepared by the government.

The agencies that responded to my request included the Department of Health and Human Services/Centers for Disease Control (sending 5 brochures); the Departments of Health from the states of Illinois (13), Texas (6), and Maryland (2); the San Francisco AIDS Foundation (7); the American Red Cross (3); the American College Health Association (2); the American Social Health Association (1); and ETR Associates, a California organization that produces health education literature (1). Because these brochures are addressed to several different populations, are distributed in various regions of the nation, and are produced by both government and private agencies, they are demonstrative of the type of information individuals received in an attempt to slow the spread of HIV/AIDS across the United States in the early 1990s.

After securing the brochures, I performed a textual analysis focusing on the following questions: What does the instruction/education about condom use in the brochures reveal about sexual attitudes and practices in the early 1990s? and How have attitudes, values, and beliefs concerning sexuality affected the ways in which the government and private organizations communicate about condom use?

Analysis

Acknowledging heterosexual women as individuals who may become infected with HIV was a difficult step because heterosexual women did not conveniently fit into the previously defined groups of "guilty victims" (gay men, intravenous drug [IV] users) and "innocent victims" (hemophiliacs, children). Indeed, these women were most likely infected by having sexual intercourse with an IV drug user or man who was infected with HIV; yet, by keeping them out of the "at risk" population, the general population did not have to panic too much. As is the case with all sexually transmitted diseases, AIDS offers a point in our cultural history where we may examine what Brandt (1987) has termed the rational/scientific and the behavioral/ moralistic approaches working in tandem to produce acceptable identities for those involved in the pandemic. For example, two of the brochures (*There Are Three Words Every Black Person Should Know* and *Condoms and Sexually Transmitted Diseases...Especially AIDS*) explicitly state that readers should not have anal sex. Of course, there is a rational/scientific reason for this warning: HIV is easily transmitted during anal sex. However, there is also a behavioral/moralistic judgment residing in the message: The fact that only two of the brochures explicitly tell women not to have anal sex suggests that this is an act women should not be engaging in already. When deciphering how sexual attitudes and practices are revealed via discussions about condom use and in looking at how cultural attitudes are reflected in the advice given to readers, it will be most helpful to consider the distinction between rational/scientific and behavioral/moralistic.

Educating Readers about Condom Usage

Not surprisingly, all but two of the brochures contained information about condoms. Although male condom use is featured predominantly in the brochures, 53 percent (n=20) stress that condoms, while effective, are not foolproof. A representative sample reads: "When used properly, condoms help protect you. But, they can *fail*. Not having sex is the safest" (*AIDS— Women Get It Too*, p. 5). These brochures carry with them the message that readers, mostly women, should ideally abstain from sexual intercourse altogether. In the brochure directed at gay men, however, the Illinois Department of Health asks that readers "*consider* not having sex" (p. 5, my emphasis). Perhaps the authors feel more comfortable issuing orders to women about their sex lives or are basing their advice to gay men on stereotypes that it would be more difficult for gay men to stop having sexual intercourse than heterosexual women; thus they ask only gay men to consider not having sex and do not give women the same option to make their own choices.

Given that the ultimate purpose of these brochures is to educate readers about HIV/AIDS, it is remarkable that while 95 percent of the brochures mention condoms, 50 percent (n=19) of the brochures do not provide readers with instructions about how to use condoms. Whereas 26 percent (n=10) of the brochures tell readers to use condoms properly and correctly, they fail to instruct readers how to use condoms properly. Only five brochures provide readers with written instructions for proper condom usage, and four brochures provide both illustrated and written instructions for proper condom usage. Of the four brochures that provide both written and illustrated instructions, three are produced by private organizations. This disparity suggests that the governmental agencies, which make up the majority of the brochures that offer readers no information about proper condom usage, are not doing their job to help reduce the spread of HIV because they are not informing readers about proper condom usage. The one exception is the brochure directed at gay men developed by the Illinois Department of Health. This brochure has an entire page devoted to informing readers about how to use condoms correctly and includes a discussion of the proper types of lubricants to use. It should not be too surprising that the state agency felt free to be direct and open when communicating with gay men, since they are a group that has been associated with HIV/AIDS since its inception; yet, by not being just as open and direct with women, especially when discussing proper condom usage, the authors are doing women a disservice by not helping them protect themselves.

Interestingly enough, although only one-half of the brochures mention instructions for proper condom usage, 71 percent (n=27) of the brochures tell readers that they should use a spermicide in addition to a condom to reduce the risk of becoming infected with HIV. Yet only 32 percent (n=12) of the brochures inform readers about the types of lubricants that can cause condoms to become weakened and then break.

When discussing different types of sexual intercourse and condom use, 50 percent of the brochures do not even mention that a condom should be used during different types of sexual intercourse. Fifty percent note that a condom should be used during vaginal intercourse and 45 percent of the brochures mention that condoms should be used during oral and anal intercourse. As noted above, two brochures actually tell women not to have anal sex, even with a condom, because of the risk. One brochure, produced by the U.S. Department of Health and Human Services, follows a question-and-answer format, and one of the questions reads, "Are condoms strong enough for anal sex?" The answer reads, "The Surgeon General has said, 'Condoms provide some protection, but anal intercourse is simply too dangerous a practice'" (*Condoms and Sexually Transmitted Diseases...Especially AIDS*, p. 7). Clearly, his words are meant to stop women, and other members of the general population, from having anal intercourse. The other brochure, produced by Maryland's Department of Health, notes: "We know the AIDS virus is spread by anal or rectal sex. Don't have anal sex—it's really risky" (*8 out of 10 Women*, p. 4). These brochures are the only two that go so far as to overtly recommend that readers radically modify their behavior by not having anal sex at all. Only three brochures, all published by private organizations, note that condoms should also be used with sex toys. This is telling because sex toys are not generally thought of as being "mainstream," thus the government brochures do not address the use of sex toys at all in any of their brochures.

Only one brochure, written in 1992, mentions the female condom, which at that time was undergoing FDA review. Only four brochures (11 percent), all produced by private organizations, discuss using dental dams when performing oral sex on women. As three of the four brochures are directed at lesbians, it is not surprising that cunnilingus should be discussed within this context. It is telling that women are not told about men's risk when performing oral sex on women in the other brochures; instead, the focus is on women performing oral sex on men.

One of the more fascinating instructions female readers are given involves the purchase and use of condoms. Thirteen percent (n=5) of the brochures directed at women tell readers that they should be responsible for purchasing condoms or for making sure that they have sex using condoms. One brochure tells readers, "Keep some condoms handy, in case your partner doesn't have any. You can buy condoms at the store" (*AIDS—Women Get It*

Too, p. 6). In terms of who's responsible for purchasing and making sure condoms are used during intercourse, one author writes, "Condoms are not just for men....Protection against infection with HIV is the responsibility of both you and your partner" (*Women, Sex, and HIV*, p. 7). Another states, "Make sure you have condoms with you....Don't depend on your man to have them" (*AIDS: An African American Woman's Story*, p. 5). These excerpts are positive because they may serve to empower women by encouraging them to be responsible for the purchasing of condoms and, by extension, their own sexual identities. Two other brochures discuss the difficulty women may have when trying to get their partners to use condoms during sexual intercourse: "It's hard for some women to talk with their men about sex and using condoms. But telling your man to wear a rubber doesn't mean you don't trust him. It's not about trust—it's about love. Love for life, love for him, and love of yourself" (*8 out of 10 Women*, p. 3) and "Right now the most effective way to prevent AIDS besides not having sex is a condom. Even though you might not want to use one—or even though *he* might not want to use one, learn how. And learn how to use them properly. Your life may depend on it" (*There Are Three Words Every Black Person Should Know*, p. 2). The previous examples depend on emotional appeals for the reader to comply with the prescribed behavior. This strategy is more typical and does not grant women much agency per se. In these excerpts, women are expected to be able to articulate their desire for their partner to use a condom but are not given specific strategies to help them enact this goal. In the only instance when condom purchases are mentioned in brochures directed at the general population, a young Caucasian man is pictured holding a box of condoms and talking to an older Caucasian man, presumably a pharmacist. This image reinforces the notion that men are the ones who regularly purchase the condoms. Given that this stereotype is only challenged in brochures addressed to women, it may hurt women's reputations if they are the ones who produce condoms prior to sexual intercourse, especially since the brochures targeted to the general population say nothing about who should purchase condoms or anything about condom usage being the responsibility of both men and women.

When attempting to educate readers about condom usage in an attempt to slow the spread of HIV, the government brochures are at best vague and at worst harmful because readers, especially women, are not getting the necessary information that they need to protect themselves from being infected with HIV.

Persuading Readers to Use Condoms

When evaluating the persuasive strategies utilized to try and get readers to use condoms during sexual intercourse, a few authors approach readers in an empowering way. Some readers are told that condom use will serve to enhance their sexual experiences: "Condoms can make sex better. Sometimes sex lasts longer if he's wearing a condom. Condoms can be a great part of sex play if you know how to use them" (*8 out of 10 Women*, p. 3); "*You* put it on. Make it fun—a part of foreplay" (*AIDS: An African American Woman's Story*, p. 6); "Using condoms can be sexy. Ask your partner for help putting them on" (*What Men in the Gay Community Should Know About AIDS*, p. 7); "You can still feel the heat. You can touch, look at, and smell her. The only thing you are giving up is the taste" (*Safer Sex Handbook for Lesbians*, p. 3); and "They're [condoms are] inexpensive, easy to buy and carry and they can be fun to use!" (*AIDS ABCs*, p. 1). It is telling that only one of the five brochures that discuss condoms as enhancing sexual intercourse is directed to the general population. The other brochures are targeted to women of color, lesbians, and gay men. This implies that the general population should not be persuaded to use condoms because they will enhance pleasure. This is distressing not only because other women are not receiving the potentially empowering message that condoms may enhance pleasure associated with sexual intercourse, but also because it suggests that other women need not enjoy sexual intercourse, or at the very least, they do not need to know this benefit of condom use.

While all of the brochures exert a rational/scientific approach when discussing HIV/AIDS and, implicitly, offer a behavioral/moralistic approach by prescribing behaviors that will keep readers "safer," few authors discuss how women should communicate about condom use with their partner. Here is one example of the information readers encounter:

> **Talk to your partner *before* you have sex.** Be honest in talking about AIDS: Pick a time when you're both relaxed. Let your partner know your concerns. Listen to your partner. Don't accuse your partner of anything. Plan what to say if your partner refuses to use a latex condom. Insist on using one. Do it for your sake—and for those you love. (*AIDS—Women Get It Too*, p. 6)

This excerpt is interesting because it instructs women to not accuse their partners of anything and does not give any specific strategies to get their partners to use condoms. Moreover, this brochure does not discuss the consequences if a woman insists on using a condom and her partner refuses.

Another example reads:

> "**How can I talk to my partner about 'safer sex'?**" Pick a time when you can talk freely and without interruption. Be honest, and admit your concerns. Don't give in to pressure—insist on what protects both of you." (*About AIDS and Shooting Drugs*, p. 14)

This author suggests that readers, in this case both men and women, stress that they are helping their partners as well as themselves.

Two brochures, both directed at African-American women, acknowledge the difficulty inherent in women discussing issues surrounding sexual intercourse. One brochure states:

> **Talk to Him.** It's hard for some women to talk with their men about sex and using condoms. But telling your man to wear a rubber doesn't mean you don't trust him. It's not about trust—it's about love. Love for life, love for him and love of yourself....More and more women are telling their men to wear condoms. And more and more men do. Don't you think it's a good idea? (*8 out of 10 Women*, p. 4)

This excerpt is significant because it acknowledges that more and more women are telling, not asking, but telling their men to wear condoms. In addition, the authors provide women with a communication strategy within the excerpt: When women ask that their partners wear condoms, they are not saying they do not trust them, they are saying that they love their partners and themselves and wish to keep on living. The other brochure that acknowledges the difficulty of women discussing sexual intercourse is much more prescriptive:

> **How Do I Discuss Safe Sex with My Partner?** First of all, learn as much as you can about AIDS. Second, be frank. AIDS kills, so the thing you don't want to do is put yourself at risk. If you have oral, anal, or vaginal sex with an infected person, chances are you will become infected too. That means man to woman, woman to man, man to man, woman to woman, all of it! And because there is no cure, we all must work at preventing its spread. Right now, the most effective way to prevent AIDS besides not having sex is a condom. Even though you might not want to use one—or even though *he* might not want to use one, learn how. And learn to use them properly. Your life may depend on it. (*There Are Three Words Every Black Person Should Know*, p. 2)

This advice is unique because it invites female readers to put themselves first. As is often the case in these brochures, women's needs and lives are second to others; however, one of the first things this author acknowledges is that women should not want to put their own lives at risk.

Another pamphlet directed at African-American women, entitled *AIDS: An African American Woman's Story*, alerts readers to their possible fate if they do not convince their partners to use a condom during sexual intercourse. This pamphlet focuses on a woman named "Tanya" and her experiences with HIV and eventually AIDS. Tanya's sister narrates the brochure and tells readers that Tanya became infected with HIV by her boyfriend, Jamal, who was an IV drug user. Tanya tells her sister, "I tried to get Jamal to use a condom. But he got mad. He said I didn't trust him. I was so afraid of losing him that I just gave in. Now I wish I had respected myself more. Then I would have stood up to Jamal" (p. 3). This is an effective example because it asks readers to identify with a specific individual who is now HIV-positive and, by the end of the pamphlet, dies from AIDS. Later, Tanya tells her sister, "And if he refuses to use a condom, you tell him—sorry, no glove, no love" (p. 5). While this is an empowering statement, one wonders how realistic it is. Will men abide by this choice? Is it acceptable for women to simply say, "No glove, no love?" What are the consequences when women insist that their partners use condoms?

Only one pamphlet out of the entire sample addresses issues of abuse and domestic violence women may encounter when taking charge of their own sex lives and practices. The brochure, entitled *Women, Sex, and HIV*, includes the following statement:

> Talking about safer sex methods may be impossible if you are in an abusive or violent relationship. Raising sensitive subjects like HIV may increase tension. If you cannot talk about HIV or using protection without having a fight, consider seeking help from a counselor or someone else who can help with relationship problems. Check your local yellow pages directory or call your local public health department for information about shelter for battered or abused women in your area. (p. 8)

This excerpt is particularly useful for readers because it offers them direction while acknowledging the fact that not all women are able to talk with their partners about condom use or even HIV/AIDS without being threatened.

Overall, the brochures published by the government do not adequately inform readers about proper condom use, completely ignore the need to use a dental dam when individuals perform oral sex on women, encourage African-American women to use condoms because they may enhance sexual intercourse, provide no specific examples for readers to follow when trying to persuade their partners to use a condom during sexual intercourse, and do not realistically address the position women may be in when discussing their sex lives and practices with their partners. This suggests that when speaking to the general population, issues surrounding sexuality are to be treated in a vague, yet appropriate, manner despite the fact that the information is being distributed in an attempt to save lives. The government's puritanical approach when discussing sexuality with the general population seems to fade when communicating to women of color and to gay men. This contradiction, as discussed below, can both help and harm these groups of individuals.

Conclusion
When reviewing the HIV/AIDS brochures targeted at women and produced by governmental agencies at the beginning of the early 1990s, a clear dichotomy surfaces: Brochures directed at the general population (i.e., Caucasian women) use "proper" scientific language and include very vague and brief discussions of condom usage, whereas brochures directed at women of color use slang (e.g., condoms are referred to as "rubbers" and semen is called "cum") and contain a lengthier discussion about condom usage. This difference ultimately places women of color in a double bind; these brochures assist women of color by identifying them as a population at risk of becoming infected with HIV, but the brochures also stigmatize these women by identifying them with the HIV/AIDS pandemic.

What is perhaps most telling is the difference in tone and language between the brochures produced by governmental agencies and those produced by private organizations. Given the fact that no governmental agencies developed brochures to alert lesbians to their risk of becoming infected with HIV, it seems that governmental agencies are working under constraints as to the types of populations they can address. In addition, the pamphlets produced by private organizations are much more direct, filled with more helpful information, and seem as if they would be more acceptable to readers given their direct tone and clear instructions. In looking at the brochures published when women's HIV identities were first being developed, it is not surprising that women continue to be the fastest-growing population to be infected with HIV. These brochures, while not representative of the entire cultural response to HIV/AIDS, fail to recognize the obstacles women face when they try to communicate about safer sex and ultimately reclaim their sexuality by demanding that their partners use condoms. Instead, the brochures produced by governmental agencies pacify the general population with a generic discussion of HIV/AIDS while alerting a small minority of women that they may be at risk. Ultimately, these brochures failed to accomplish their task because readers were not provided with clear communicative strategies to combat some cultural views that women should not be too direct when talking about sexual intercourse or even when having sexual intercourse.

Bibliography

Brandt, A. M. (1987). *No magic bullet: A social history of venereal disease in the United States since 1880.* Oxford: Oxford University Press.

Centers for Disease Control. (2000a). Basic statistics: International statistics. Retrieved August 18, 2000, from the Internet: *www.cdc.gov/hiv/stats/internat.html.*

Centers for Disease Control. (2000b). HIV/AIDS among U.S. women: Minority and young women at continuing risk. Retrieved August 18, 2000, from the Internet: *www.cdcnpin.org/news/updates.html.*

Centers for Disease Control. (1993a). U.S. department of health and human services, food and drug administration. Retrieved June 20, 2002, from the Internet: *www.aegis.com/pubs/CDC_Fact_Sheets/1993/CDC93033. html.*

Centers for Disease Control. (1993b). Women's interagency HIV study begins. Retrieved June 20, 2002, from the Internet: *www.aegis.com/pubs/ CDC_Fact_Sheets/1993/CDC93039.html.*

National Institute of Allergy and Infectious Diseases. (2004). HIV infection in women. Retrieved March 15, 2005 from the Internet: *www.niaid.nih. gov/factsheets/womenhiv.htm.*

National Institutes of Health. (2002). HIV/AIDS statistics. Retrieved June 20, 2002 from the Internet: *www.niaid.nih.gov/factsheets/aidsstat.htm.*

Brochures Used for Analysis:

American College Health Association. (1990). *HIV infection and AIDS: What everyone should know.*

American College Health Association. (1990). *Women and AIDS.*

American Red Cross. (1988). *Women, sex, and AIDS*.

American Red Cross. (1990). *Testing for HIV infection*.

American Red Cross. (1992). *Women, sex, and HIV*.

American Social Health Association. (1992). *Positive living*.

Centers for Disease Control. (No date). *There are three words every black person should know: AIDS doesn't discriminate*.

ETR Associates. (1989). *AIDS ABCs*.

Illinois Department of Public Health. (1985). *What gay and bisexual men should know about AIDS*.

Illinois Department of Public Health. (1987). *What everyone should know about AIDS*.

Illinois Department of Public Health. (1991). *About AIDS and shooting drugs*.

Illinois Department of Public Health. (1991). *Anyone can get AIDS*.

Illinois Department of Public Health. (1991). *Getting married? Know the facts about your sexual health*.

Illinois Department of Public Health. (1992). *I'm not living in the dark anymore. Why are you? AIDS: See the light*.

Illinois Department of Public Health. (1992). *What men in the gay community should know about AIDS*.

Illinois Department of Public Health. (1993). *AIDS antibody testing*.

Illinois Department of Public Health. (1993). *AIDS—Women get it too*.

Illinois Department of Public Health. (1993). *Is someone giving you something you don't want?*

Illinois Department of Public Health. (1994). *AIDS: Facts for teens.*

Illinois Department of Public Health. (1994). *Their past could make you history.*

Illinois Department of Public Health. (1994). *Why you should be informed about AIDS.*

Maryland Department of Health and Mental Hygiene. (1992). *8 out of 10 women with AIDS are women of color.*

Maryland Department of Health and Mental Hygiene. (1995). *AIDS: An African American woman's story.*

Texas Department of Public Health. (1991). *AIDS and the workplace.*

Texas Department of Public Health. (1992). *AIDS and the injecting drug user.*

Texas Department of Public Health. (1993). *AIDS/HIV and the African American community.*

Texas Department of Public Health. (1993). *HIV/AIDS and women.*

Texas Department of Public Health. (1993). *Should you get an HIV test?*

Texas Department of Public Health. (1993). *What everyone should know about AIDS.*

San Francisco AIDS Foundation. (1991). *AIDS and lesbians.*

San Francisco AIDS Foundation. (1992). *AIDS family guide: Responding with your heart.*

San Francisco AIDS Foundation. (1992). *AIDS kills women and babies.*

San Francisco AIDS Foundation. (1992). *Pregnancy and HIV.*

San Francisco AIDS Foundation. (1992). *Women and HIV.*

San Francisco AIDS Foundation. (1993). *Safer sex handbook for lesbians.*

San Francisco AIDS Foundation. (1994). *Living with HIV: A guide for women.*

U.S. Department of Health and Human Services. (1991). *Condoms and sexually transmitted diseases . . . especially AIDS.*

U.S. Department of Health and Human Services. (1991). *HIV infection and AIDS: Are you at risk?*

U.S. Department of Health and Human Services. (1993). *Voluntary HIV counseling and testing: Facts, issues, and answers.*

U.S. Department of Health and Human Services. (1994). *HIV and your child.*

Willis, J. L. (1997). *Equality in clinical trials: Drugs and gender.* Retrieved March 16, 2005 from the Internet: *www.fda.gov/oashi/aids/ equal.html*

• CHAPTER TWELVE •

Female Identity and the Construction of Condom Use Among Young African-American Women

Janis Faye Hutchinson

Heterosexual contact is currently the most reported avenue for HIV infection among women. There are three major reasons that women in the United States are at higher risk, compared with men, of encountering an HIV-infected heterosexual partner. First, most intravenous drug users and virtually all hemophiliacs are men. Second, sexual partners of some women are bisexuals (the number is unknown) who contract it through sexual contact with other men. Third, some studies suggest that male to female transmission is easier than female to male (Ellerbrock et al., 1991; Padian, Shiboski, & Jewell, 1991).

Condom use, mutual monogamy, treatment for other sexually transmitted infections (STIs), and partner reduction are emphasized in AIDS prevention programs to control the spread of HIV (Ananth & Koopman, 2003; Geary, Tchupo, & Johnson, 2003; Gupta & Weiss, 1993; Ku, Sonenstein, & Pleck, 1994; Soet, Dilorio, & Dudley, 1998 However, despite the risk of HIV and other STIs, most surveys show inconsistent condom use. That is, studies indicate that women and men do not practice protective behaviors such as reducing the number of sex partners (Grinstead et al., 1993; Leigh, Temple, & Trocki, 1993; Reinisch et al., 1992; Richens, Imrie, & Copas, 2000, Sawyer & Moss, 1993) and using condoms (Amirkhanian, Kelly, & Kabakchieva, 2003; Camlin & Chimbwete, 2003; Catania et al., 1994; Kost and Forrest, 1992; Soet et al., 1998). It has been reported that only a third of sexually active women and men use condoms with their regular partners, and consistent condom use ranges between 10 and 20 percent (Catania et al., 1994; Radcliffe et al., 1993). The non-use of condoms is not related to lack of knowledge about STIs, especially HIV transmission (Catania et al., 1992; Mays & Cochran, 1988; Selwyn et al., 1989) or lack of knowledge about the consequences of infection (Gupta & Mahy, 2001; Pivnick, 1993).

A variety of issues have been examined to explain inconsistent condom use. Most studies that investigate condom use examine attitudinal characteristics that affect condom use (Jemmott & Jemmott, 1991; Ku et al., 1994;

Lollis et al., 1996; Wiggers, de Wit, & Gras, 2003) such as intrapersonal predictors of men's condom use (Johnson et al., 1992; Pleck, Sonenstein, & Ku, 1990) and intrapersonal predictors of condom use among women in comparison to men (Gupta & Weiss, 1993; O'Leary et al., 1992; Wulfert & Wan, 1993). Interpersonal predictors of condom use have been examined among college women (Gupta & Weiss, 1993; Hinkle et al., 1992) and indicate the importance of sociocultural factors such as gender roles, socialization, and power in relationships that relate to ethnic variation (Giffin, 1998; Holland et al., 1990, 1992; Soet et al., 1998). Gender issues in condom use have been mostly examined among women at high risk for infection such as injection drug users (Kline, Kline, & Oken, 1992; Pivnick, 1993; Worth, 1989), women in high-risk settings such as clinic populations (Detzer et al., 1995; Sobo, 1993; Upchurch et al., 1992) and among adolescents (Moore & Rosenthal, 1991). There is a paucity of studies examining black women and condom use outside of traditional high-risk groups (Cummings et al, 1997; Flaskerud & Nyamthi, 1989; Flaskerud & Rush, 1989; Jemmott & Jemmott, 1991).

It is assumed, usually mistakenly, that when people consider using condoms they are making a rational decision (Worth, 1989). Such studies have not considered the gendered nature of sexual behavior or cultural values and norms. In particular, an assumption in models of sexual behaviors is that encounters are controlled by the individual (Amaro, 1995). However, the current study suggests social costs that affect women's ability to negotiate condom use. In the current study, the meaning of condom use was examined among young adult African-American women who deny risks for HIV and other STIs.

METHODS

The data were collected in two parts. The first part of the study was qualitative in scope and involved intensive interviews. These interviews provided the contextual background for the exploration of condom use among young adult African-American women in Houston. The second phase of the study was a quantitative analysis that provided information on the prevalence of beliefs, attitudes, and behaviors associated with condom use in this population.

Research Site

African-American women were solicited at a local gangsta rap nightclub (Club X, fictitious name) in Houston, Texas, between 1993 and 1997. This nightclub is not unique among black nightclubs in Houston. It is similar to other black nightclubs in terms of age and sex composition and percentage of nonwhites (small numbers of whites and Hispanics). However, it is different in terms of the greater amount of gangsta rap music played at the nightclub. Gangsta rap is the controversial type of music that you may hear about in the local news. These rappers espouse themes of killing and use of guns and make extremely derogatory statements about women and explicit sexual statements. The music also portrays realistic views of life in the African-American community and what it is like to be black in a white-dominated American society. This music appeals to diverse groups of younger African Americans. Other nightclubs for younger adults play some gangsta rap, but the majority of the music can be classified as other types of rap, reggae, and rhythm and blues. Nightclub X was chosen because many young African Americans frequent this club and because a former student introduced me to the types of activities that occur at and near the nightclub. The student was infected with HIV by one of the "regulars" at the club. Through discussions with her, I learned about sexual transactions in her network and that this nightclub was a focal point for their sexual interactions.

Intensive Interviews

Women were approached between 1993 and 1995 about taking part in the intensive interviews. They were approached in the restroom and if they agreed to participate, I recorded their names and telephone numbers. Later, I telephoned each and set up an appointment for an interview. Five African-American women between the ages of 22 and 32 who frequented Nightclub X were intensively interviewed. Women were very diverse in terms of their backgrounds. For example, LaQuita was a 28-year-old female with 3 children. She did not finish high school and did not have a GED. LaQuita had her first child at 17 and was unemployed and on welfare. She said she wanted to go to school but did not have a babysitter or job. Shontele was a 25-year-old female with one child who lived with her parents. She had a boyfriend, but he left her for another woman. Latasha was a 22-year-old college student with no children. She lived with her mother and had been with her boyfriend for 4 years. Anna was a 32-year-old professional working woman with no children. Yvonne was a 25-year-old college student with no children. She dated a number of men, many of whom were drug dealers. She became

HIV-seropositive during the time period discussed in this paper. (Note: All names are fictitious.)

Topics discussed in intensive interviews dealt with sexism, love/romance, fidelity, economics, and reasons for condom use/non-use. These interview topics were based on the literature and informal interviews with women at the nightclub. The interviews consisted of open-ended discussions that allowed participants to venture into areas not specifically outlined in the protocol. In this way, cultural themes, "elements in the patterns that make up a culture," were identified (Spradley, 1980, p. 14). Cultural themes usually take the form of an assertion that is highly generalizable (Spradley, 1980). In the interviews, assertions were usually followed by examples. Themes were given labels, and patterns and trends were identified. While intensive interview data does not provide insights into the prevalence of attitudes and behaviors, it does give insights into the context of behavioral patterns. Interviews lasted between one and a half and four hours and were conducted at the participants' homes, the biocultural laboratory at the University of Houston, a park, and a McDonald's restaurant. Interviews were tape recorded and transcribed verbatim by a professional. Interviewees were given a small monetary compensation.

Selection and Recruitment for the Survey
The survey component took place between September 1996 and August 1997. African-American women between the ages of 18 and 35 years who frequented Nightclub X were recruited for the survey. After "hanging out" at the nightclub to recruit women for the intensive interview component, people were used to seeing me and some knew that I was doing a study on male/female relationships. I went to the restroom periodically to solicit people for the study. I waited for a large crowd, because if one person agreed, an additional two or more would participate. I went back and forth to the restroom and each time explained the study to the group present. If they agreed to participate, I recorded their names and telephone numbers. Later, I called and set up an appointment to interview them. The snowball sampling technique was also used to recruit additional people. These individuals were friends of those interviewed and frequented Nightclub X (N=50; Response Rate=35%). Interviews lasted one to two hours and took place at people's homes, the biocultural laboratory, and restaurants. At the time of the interview, more details on the purpose of the survey were explained and, if the person agreed to participate, the consent form was signed. A face-to-face

survey was then administered. Interviewees were given a small monetary compensation.

The survey covered demographics, sexual activity, condom use, importance of marriage, family, and sexism. Sections and items on the survey were based on content analysis of intensive interviews and a review of the literature on condom use and male/female relationships.

The survey was pilot-tested for understandability in a sample of ten African-American women during the summer of 1996. The women were African-American students and staff at the University of Houston and were recruited through the snowball technique. They ranged in age from 24 to 49 years old.

The average age of women in the survey was 24.44 years (sd=3.15) with an age range of 19–35 years. The majority of the women were single (86%). Over half of the participants had some college education (54%), 3% were college graduates, 25% were high school graduates, and 17% had less than a high school education. Many were also employed (76%) and had worked during the past six months (72%). Their occupations were usually low-wage work such as clerical, fast food, and day care. Most of the women did not have children (58%); 30% had one child, 10% had two children, and 2% had three children.

RESEARCH FINDINGS

Committed and Casual Relationships

At the beginning of a relationship, women reported using condoms. However, once the relationship was considered monogamous, condoms were discontinued. The following are examples of this theme.

Latasha and her boyfriend did not use condoms, although he carried them in his pocket. Latasha said:

> I'm concerned. I'm very concerned. We don't use condoms. But you know, he carries them, which is fine. You know the thought that he carries them is good, but then it's not good, because, you know. But we don't. The reason why? I just feel like because we go together, although I know we should. But I know it's really not like that. I feel that I trust him, even though in the back of my mind I know I shouldn't, but I do. I trust him. I feel old fashioned. I feel that if you're in a relationship, that's it, and we've been together off and on for four or five years. So I just feel that I trust him, and when we do date we are together. It's important, but I just don't worry about it, you know.

In addition, Shontele stopped using condoms when she and her boyfriend tested negative for HIV. After they tested negative, she said, "we decided we weren't going to use them anymore." Condoms were not considered necessary since they were HIV-negative and in a monogamous relationship.

In these examples, continued use of condoms in a long-term relationship threatened the trust implied in the relationship and suggested that the relationship would remain static (Holland et al., 1992; Worth, 1989), that is, that the relationship would remain casual and non-monogamous. The social meanings associated with condom use included transgressing constructions of intimacy and lack of fidelity and monogamy (Pivnick, 1993; Worth, 1989). When trust is implicit and monogamy is assumed between partners, condom use can be interpreted as endangering or challenging a steady relationship (Holland et al., 1992).

Even if the relationship is no longer monogamous, women still want to believe their ex-boyfriend will practice protective behaviors. For instance, LaQuita was not sure if Bob was using a condom with his new girlfriend (he was still intimate with LaQuita and they did not use condoms). "I said, 'Bob, you're having sex with this girl. Why you don't use condoms with the girl you messing with and then having sex with me?' You never know. He said, 'I'm using condoms.'" This statement was enough for LaQuita to continue unsafe sex with an ex-boyfriend. Even when the relationship was obviously non-monogamous, condoms were not used. They were not used because of the "hope" for a committed relationship.

When women have more than one boyfriend or sex partner they are more likely to use condoms. For instance, Anna used condoms with both of her lovers. With the secondary partner, they had used condoms since the beginning of the relationship. However, it was later in the relationship when she discussed it with her primary partner. In the survey, those with two or more sex partners were more likely to use condoms (21% used condoms more than half the time versus 3% less than half the time) compared to those with one partner (22% used condoms more than half the time versus 54% less than half the time). Other studies, such as Svenson, Ostergren, and Merlo (2002), found that a larger number of sex partners predicted inconsistent condom use.

Yvonne's situation was very different from that of the other women because she lived in a physically dangerous social environment. Yvonne gave the following two examples to describe her environment.

> We were in Bennigan's one night and somebody was messing with him [Lance, her boyfriend] and he kept messing with this one guy and the guy took a Long Island tea

• Female Identity and the Construction of Condom Use •   137

glass and hit Lance in the head. Well he just stood there and the guy who did it ran out the door. Lance didn't say a word but five guys ran out after him, beat him up. No one said nothing. You say to yourself, I do not want to piss these people off, but you be with them the very next day. I was not afraid that I would be hurt.

After Anthony got out of jail one day he was in Whataburger and his baby's mother was there. She was mad about something and her friend came out and hit him. She did something to him. She pissed him off so he got a bat and hit her in the head. She went to her car and got a gun and shot him in the stomach. He falls back and said [to his friend], "I'm shot in the stomach take me to the hospital." No one gets paranoid. Everyone including him was real calm. He had a lot of stitches. I know because I had sex with him while he had stitches.

In Yvonne's circle, they did not use or discuss condoms.

Lot of the time when we had sex, people were high or drunk. Never thought about what happened until you wake up in the morning. People didn't care who you had slept with before.

In terms of condom use, most respondents in the survey did not consistently use condoms. Only 28% of the respondents always used condoms, and 42% never used them. Half did not use a condom the last time they had sex (52%).

Eleven percent of the women reported rape where they were forced to have sex with men who did not use condoms. Yvonne discussed a night when her boyfriend raped her girlfriend.

I remember one night we were at Lance's house and we were changing to go to a club. He was a really sick person. He was in the tub and he said, "Tell your friend to come in here and wash my back." I said no. He got mad at me for not telling her. He got mad like that. Everything had to be the way that he wanted. He went in the room and he was getting dressed and then he left. I was in the bathroom and she was in the bedroom getting dressed. I heard him come in. But I didn't think about where he went. So I opened the bathroom door and looked around and didn't see anybody so I closed the door. I thought he had gone back out. She was still in the room. She came out of the room and he had been in the room too. I didn't know that. He said, "I'm going to go on over there and ya'll can meet me there." When we were in the car she was real quiet. I said, "Trina, what's wrong with you?" She said nothing. We get to the club and he wasn't there. She found a friend of hers and she started crying and ran out of the club. Her friend ran after her and I ran after them trying to figure out what's going on. It turned out he had been in the room with her and he had raped her. I am so lost. I really couldn't believe it. I met another girl at the club who was sitting with Trina. She was sleeping with Lance too. She went to where he was and confronted him in front of all of these people. [The friend of the girl who was raped took her home.]

It is clear that women do not consistently use condoms. The ensuing sections provide further explanations for inconsistent condom use in this sample of women.

Love/Marriage/Children

Studies indicate that love, spontaneity, and commitment to a monogamous relationship are more important than the risk of STIs such as HIV (Sobo, 1993; Worth, 1989). As such, in connection to inconsistent condom use, women reported being in love with their boyfriends and perceived a committed relationship or the hope for a committed relationship. Using condoms was contrary to their goal, a relationship. Moreover, sex is viewed as the actualization of a relationship and not as an isolated erotic activity among black females (Fullilove et al., 1990a; Heise & Elias, 1995). For this sample of women, they are not "whole" unless they are attached to a male, socially and sexually. Their sense of female identity is related to this attachment. For instance, in the intensive interviews, women continually discussed the importance of being in a relationship and "having a man." Their sense of self and well-being was related to their attachment to a man. As such, protective behaviors, such as condom use, run counter to female identity constructed in terms of committed and intimate relationships. While discussing relationships, LaQuita said, "Every woman don't want to be alone." Latasha also does not want to be alone.

> I felt like I needed a boyfriend and a best friend. I wanted him to be everything in one. For a short time he was all of that. I did whatever. If he said that something was right and my parents said it wasn't then I went with him instead of my family. He was there when I needed somebody to talk to and at one point in time I had no friends. My whole life was centered around him.

Marriage is very important to Latasha.

> I can hope that ten years from now I'm married with about five kids. And I'm just happy and I'm stable and working. Just doing home stuff. If I never get married I'd feel that I hadn't accomplished anything because I hadn't succeeded in a goal that I had planned. It's not just to be married to somebody but just that person you know is going to be special. You don't want to go through life dating forever and ever. It's not good. After a while it's boring. I don't want to be married for financial reasons but for that special person.

Although Anna planned or would like to be married by age 35, she would be happy simply to be in a relationship.

> I feel like if God didn't want me to marry anybody I can live with my mother. I wouldn't think that there would not be anyone that I was not compatible with. I would not feel that my life was a failure if I did not get married or did not have children. If I could live with somebody for the rest of my life that would be fine. We don't have to be married if we don't want to be married. Companionship is everything. Being alone and being lonely are two different things. I do enjoy being alone, though.

Eighty percent of the survey participants said it was important or very important to be married. In addition, 61% believed they must be in a relationship to have a child and 70% wanted a child. For instance, women said they wanted to have a child so they could be a mother and have a family (43%). Others said they wanted "to have a part of themselves" (20%) or they "like kids" (11%). Children and marriage are important goals for these women. Like other Americans, they have traditional values concerning marriage and family. These values, marriage/bonding, and children, help to define black womanhood and black femininity.

Infidelity

Studies show that while women are oriented toward the romantic, men are geared toward the physical and erotic (Houston, 1981; Leigh, 1989). There is a double standard where men can have sex for gratification but women should have sex only for love. In the black community, traditional sexual roles where men have sexual freedom and women are passive still operate (Fullilove et al., 1990a; Taylor et al., 1997). Women in the study did not find infidelity by men to be unexpected or a reason to end the relationship. Rather, one woman blamed herself for her boyfriend's infidelity. LaQuita said:

> They're not interested in a woman with a baby. Some men are more interested in women who are untouched, more pure and clean. Most men like women with the perfect measurements, no children, no sex or they only had a little sex, but you don't know a lot about sex. You don't have to have a mind or brain, you can be dumb, but you have the looks, the body. If I knew then what I know now my children would come a whole lot later and I wouldn't have had as much sex as I did. I'm old to him now. I'm going to be really old as far as a spouse or partner is concerned in a few years. I'm worried about that. I worry about it all the time.

She believes having sex and a child resulted in her "undesirability" as a permanent mate. She also said, "Some men is never satisfied with one woman." Another male friend of hers told her "sometimes one woman is not enough. You got to have more than one woman. The woman at home might be good and sweet but it takes more than one woman."

Latasha has seen condoms in her boyfriend's pocket, although he does not use them with her. She asked him about them.

> He just brushed it off. He really didn't have an answer, he just talked his way out of it like always. I kind of worry about it. I'm always on him about being with other females. Not that he's messing with someone. I'm just always worried about is he with somebody else or is he gonna sleep with somebody else. I worry about that a lot.

At first Shontele's boyfriend told her that he and the other girl were just friends. However, when she caught her boyfriend with another woman he told her "it was because the feeling wasn't there no more. He said, I love you but I feel different now. Now he said he was attracted to her." Shontele said she still loved him. After three weeks apart he came to her house and wanted to be friends. Since then she had talked to him over the telephone and said she would take him back because she loved him. Later he spent four nights with Shontele, then she did not see him over the weekend and he did not call her. The following week he told her that he was happy with the other girl. They are still intimate with each other, and the last time they had sex he did not use a condom although he is intimate with the other woman. "I asked him had he been using condoms with the girl and he said, 'You know I take this seriously.'" He claimed that he used condoms with the other girl and that he did not want a child right now. Shontele said that she believed him. In the present study only 28% cited lack of trust as a reason to use condoms. Condoms are not used even when trust has collapsed and the relationship is obviously fragile.

LaQuita recently discovered that Bob was seeing another woman. One day he would not say that he loved her over the telephone, so she went to his house.

> I go over there, knock on the door. Knock, knock, knock and it cracked open by itself. This is about 3:00 in the morning now. I went in. I pull the cover up, she raised her head up and I turned the light on. He cussed me out for coming over there. He told me he don't want to be with me no more. I was like damned. Last week you told me you know we're trying to make things work. He said I lied. This is a 360 he had done.

• Female Identity and the Construction of Condom Use • 141

That following week Bob spent the weekend with LaQuita. She thinks his new girlfriend was out of town. "That Tuesday I guess he got in touch with her and I hadn't seen him since then. It's like a 360. He said he was happy with our life. What was wrong? It's nothing. It's not you, it's me. He said he still love and care about me. I said how can you still love and care about me when you're not happy. He said feelings just don't go away that easy." LaQuita said it is

> hard to say no, you can't come over here. I do want to see him. It's hard to say no when you're in love. It's hard to say, no you can't kiss me. That's how it is when you're in love. That's how weak you get when you're in love. If he's in my face it's hard for me to say no. If we're on the phone, no. Face-to-face is hard.

LaQuita believes that all men have more than one woman because it takes more than one woman to satisfy a man. She said, "Sometimes you lose the attraction. You don't lose the feelings for the person you're with, but there's something different."

Latasha said, "Now I realize they're going to move on when they get tired of you. Some men get tired of one woman and can move on. Some men hold onto that same woman forever and still have other women." It seems that it is more important to be with him and worry than not to be with him.

> I'm trying to make him somebody that I want to spend the rest of my life with, I guess. It's hard because you try to change them but you try to take their ways and make the best of it. I don't want to be with someone else. It's hard to have another sex partner again. It's hard to move on and go be with someone else. (Latasha)

The findings of Sobo (1995) suggested a positive correlation between unsafe sex and women's feeling of insecurity about their conjugal relations. Women without jobs and those forced to rely on relationships with men, rather than extra-conjugal networks for self-esteem, were less likely to practice safe sex.

While continual introduction of condoms into a long-term relationship threatens the trust implied in such relationships, commitment to a relationship may diminish over time (Worth, 1989). Consequently, reopening the decision to use condoms may decline over time because the women are trying to reestablish a commitment that does not exist. Women deny the possibility of adultery to reduce the experience of pain and loss of status. They have difficulty telling themselves that the man they chose lies to them and is using them as a sex object (Sobo, 1993). Being cheated on by your boyfriend not only brings shame but tarnishes your sense of self.

Double standards allow men to have sex for gratification, while women can have sex only with men considered fit for a stable relationship. At the same time, women believe they should be able to identify men who are promiscuous and potentially HIV-infected (Sobo, 1993). Unsafe sex is preferable to lowering one's self-esteem by dealing with their inability to identify promiscuous or HIV-infected men—even if it means risking HIV infection.

In terms of Anna's secondary partner:

> He does have a girlfriend. And I have had boyfriends. Our relationship is based on just going to bed and sweating and that's it. There's no love and there's no commitment. We're good friends. We talk about a lot of things.

With her secondary boyfriend, "there's no jealousy, there's no emotion in this relationship. Our primary goal is to make each other happy. I don't think we would last two years if we went through that 'I don't want you seeing him and I don't want you seeing her,' it's not like that." In terms of male promiscuity, Anna said that if she caught her primary boyfriend cheating she would "kick him to the curb." According to Holland and associates (1992) empowered women may negotiate the relationship and thereby increase trust. However, intimacy produced through discussion and negotiation may obscure risks and lead to increased risk-taking in sexual relationships. This may be the case with Anna, because she takes risks with her primary boyfriend. She sees him only two to four times a month, but she still considers it a committed relationship. She had difficulty discussing what he does and whom he is with when she does not see him. Anna negotiated the relationship with her primary partner in a way that obscured her risk and increased her sexual risk-taking.

Yvonne had dated Lance for a number of years. He had previously been in prison for counterfeiting money, but at the time of the interview, he had been out for six months. She did not consider his incarceration to place her at risk for HIV infection. (It was not until later that she found out he has AIDS. At least one other person that Yvonne was intimate with is also HIV-positive.) Women do not consider unprotected sex that occurs in prisons to place them at risk, because they assume their mate is not homosexual. (The three fathers of LaQuita's children were in prison at the time of the study.) It has been shown that more women with an incarcerated partner reported never using condoms (71%) compared to those without an incarcerated partner (63%) (Cummings et al., 1997). They are not aware that 25% of black men between the ages of 20 and 29 years old are incarcerated (Russell, Wilson, & Hall, 1993) and that 30% of inmate deaths are attributed to AIDS (U.S. Department of Justice, 1993).

In the early 1990s, Yvonne and her friends did not think that their boyfriends having sex with men would harm them.

> We hung out with transsexuals, transvestites, or whatever who would dress up as women. We'd hang out with them and they all would do whatever to pay for drugs. This guy named Sun who performed at a club in the third ward and we would go see him and we'd go out afterward. This was after I broke up with Lance or we broke up with each other or whatever. I was talking about Lance because I still liked him. He must of broke up with me because I was trying to get him back. And he said, "Girl, Lance got a big dick." I said, "What you talking about?" He said, "You know I know because me and him did this and did that." I said okay and I didn't believe him because I said whatever Sun so we kind of let it go but he kept on talking about it. I said you did not and he said yes I did, yes I did. So I asked him. I said, "Lance, Sun said ya'll kind of got busy one night" or whatever. He got mad at me because I said that. He went and found Sun and they got into a fight.

> Guys would have sex with drug dealers. It was the exchange of sex for drugs. Everything had to do with sex but had to be homosexual sex not heterosexual sex. Didn't think about drug dealers having sex with the male drug addicts. We didn't think about the drug dealers we were sleeping with were the same ones having anal sex with the men drug addicts.

> Black men don't see having sex with men as homosexual. It's a bartering system. You want this from me so I'm going to get something from you. They don't do it because they want to, they do it because they want to humiliate whoever wants the crack. They want to see this man yell or scream or cry or whatever. It's funny to them. It will be about five or six of them standing around. They could care less about a person's feelings.

That same night that Lance raped Yvonne's girlfriend, the following episode occurred.

> I went back into the club and was telling Lance's best friend Rico what happened. He said, "You need to leave him alone." At the same time he was saying, "Let's eat breakfast." Me and Rico ended up at a motel that his mom owned. Well, about 4:00 in the morning we were both asleep and then there was knocking on the door. It was Lance knocking on the door with a girl named Shirley. I said, "Don't let him in, just call him on the phone." I guess Lance got mad, because Rico wouldn't let him in the room, and started banging on the door. They ended up getting a room right next door to ours. Mind you, my car is in the parking lot. He never saw my car. Rico said, "I'll call him." And I ended up leaving. That was the scariest thing and I ended up leaving. He would have been mad at me for being with his best friend. It didn't

matter that he was with another girl because he would have said I couldn't find you or something. He would have come up with something.

Lance does not hide his infidelity and expects Yvonne to accept his sex life. When Lance began dating another woman, Yvonne became friends with the woman "so I would always know where he was. So on weekends I would say come on and go out with me. That way she wouldn't be with him, not that he would be with me but he wouldn't be with her either. She and I still don't speak to this day."

At least two of the men that Yvonne dated were HIV-seropositive. Yvonne stated that she did not know that they were positive at the time they had sex because people did not talk about STIs or their sexual past. However, sometimes one's sexual past brought prestige and status. For instance, Yvonne stated:

> If I broke up with a guy and date their friend it really pisses them off. I dated Rico and he would ask me and did ya'll do it this way or that way. They'd ask and I'd say let's do it like this or like that. They'd say like damn when did you do it like that? Well when I was with so-and-so. Somebody would say, well, I know you used to date Lance. I know ya'll used to do some freaky stuff. Say yah we used to do some stuff. Automatically you get this person in your corner because you told them and they're impressed. So they want to see if it's true and have the experience too.

Because of the importance of male/female relationships, infidelity is not grounds for ending a relationship or practicing safer sex. The reason is that male-female relationships through marriage or committed or casual dating are a component of black female identity. Without this attachment, women do not think of themselves as complete. Black female identity, especially in a low-income environment, entails women attaching themselves in some way to men.

Power in Relationships
Imbalance in power between men and women can serve as a barrier to condom use. For instance, among women, sexual identity is constructed in a way that defines sex in terms of men's needs and drives. Women, then, are passive receptacles for men's passions (Holland et al., 1990). "Young women are encouraged to attach themselves socially to young men in order to succeed as conventionally feminine women, but they are then inhibited from seeing this desired and expected relationship as a structurally unequal one" (Holland et al., 1990, p. 340). It is difficult for women to negotiate condom

use when they do not expect to assert their own sexual needs and their own safety (Holland et al., 1990; Holland et al., 1992).

Besides, women's ability to negotiate condom use is dependent on male responses (Gupta & Weiss, 1993). In other words, men wear condoms, but women must persuade men to wear condoms (Amaro, 1995). However, men are conditioned by sociocultural norms that give priority to their pleasure and control in sexual relationships (Gupta & Weiss, 1993). In addition, while females can influence condom use decisions, providing condoms is the expected role of males. Consequently, males have greater control in negotiating preventive sexual behaviors (Sacco et al., 1993).

Women are also reticent to discuss condoms because it suggests they are sexually active and seeking sex. This is contrary to traditional normative behavior in which women should assume a passive sexual role, and it can result in loss of social status and sexual desirability (Worth, 1989; Worth & Rodriguez, 1987). This was suggested by LaQuita's belief that having a child resulted in her losing status as a desirable mate.

In the current study, usually both partners made the decision to use or not use a condom (73%), while women made the decision 24% of the time (men made the decision only 3% of the time). Other studies reported lack of power in sexual decision making concerning condom use (Worth, 1989), but the current study indicated that women can negotiate condom use. Rather, they do not want men to use condoms because it would threaten the relationship by suggesting extra-relationship activity and a non-monogamous, noncommitted relationship. Simultaneously, a woman claiming that she made the decision not to use condoms or that it was a dual decision may be recasting unsafe sex as an action that was chosen to reduce feelings of powerlessness. Such a claim can hide social, emotional, and economic reliance on men while indicating commitment to a fragile relationship (Sobo, 1993).

Women in intensive interviews discussed power in relationships. For instance, when asked about control in relationships, LaQuita made the following statement.

> I figure if you know how to do it you can work it. If a man can satisfy you they have the upper hand because they know you want it [sex]. If a man is good in bed, then he has control. Men have control because they have more money. For women, if you don't have that car and job they don't want you. Men are the same way. Whoever has those things can be in control. If the man is good in bed, it's hard to say who has control. They may be controlling each other.

Shontele acknowledged that relationships are related to power. "Most men have the upper hand. If a man is good in bed then he can control the woman." However, "women can control a man just like men can control a woman." Both can control the other with money and a car, but men are usually the ones with both.

> Sometimes a man might be with a woman who don't have it and they see another girl who have it. That's going to attract them and pull them on to because that girl you're with, yeah, you love and care about her, but she doesn't have that car, she doesn't have that house or that apartment or that job. Girls are the same way. If you don't have a car or a job it's good-bye. The one who has those things is in control. (LaQuita)

Latasha contended that men have power in the relationship because women want to have a man.

> I think a lot of times from what I know, uh, it's man power. Some men have power over women in the sexual area, because that woman wants to please that man and you know to hold onto that man you have to deal with what pleases him. It's important because of the relationship. You think in terms of lifelong, forever, future just relationship with this guy. You try to do whatever pleases him to hold on to him and keep him satisfied. Really, in the end, when he gets tired of you he goes on to the next. Your mind works like that and it's just now and right now. You really don't think of later on.

And, according to Yvonne, "women feel they must have unprotected sex with their boyfriends or they will date someone else." Yvonne said, "They have the status to say, 'Well, if not, see you.' They can go to the next person. Everything has to be exactly the way he says all the time."

Risky sexual behavior may occur because women perceive threats to their economic and social survival (Worth, 1989). Under- and unemployed African Americans may find sexuality a means of demonstrating womanhood. This is accomplished by having children and being sexually active in order to cope with inequalities in U.S. society, while simultaneously trying to attain a sense of achievement, creativity, and belonging (Fullilove et al., 1990b).

Women want to keep their male partners because they "don't want to be alone" and need to find a husband. Because a woman's social and economic status is determined by the male she is associated with, women may not assert any wishes that may end a relationship (Leonard, 1980). Therefore, in male-female relationships, the nonuse of condoms is related to male dominance and the woman's perception that she needs male protection, resources, and an identity that is provided through relations with her male partner (Pivnick, 1993). Since women perceive male authority and dominance over them, negotiation of condom use that is in their best interest may be considered a fruitless effort if women anticipate that men will use their power to get their way (Holland et al., 1990, 1992).

While women want to be married or in a relationship, they discussed the scarcity of black men. Sixty-four percent said that men are in short supply. Social forces, as well as environmental and institutional factors, contribute to black men becoming a population at risk. These forces include over-representation of black males in prisons, discriminatory judicial practices, poor education, unemployment, underemployment, and inadequate health care (White & Parham, 1990).

The declining economic condition of black males has been cited as a causative factor in the decline in marriage/bonding. The decline in the industrial sector, which provided employment for black men without higher education, has resulted in black males being less attractive as potential husbands and has also made them less confident that they could financially support a family (Darity & Myers, 1987; Wilson, 1987). Another economic explanation of marital decline is the growing disparity between black female and male income levels and increased economic independence of women. Research indicates that the most economically independent black women, those most highly educated, are more likely to marry than less-educated women (Taylor et al., 1997).

Women also discussed the easy availability of women compared with men. There is a gender imbalance among whites and blacks, but not Hispanics. For example, the sex ratio in 1991 was 100:100 among Hispanics, 95:100 among whites, and 88:100 for African Americans. This scarcity of men is more marked among young, sexually active age groups. The sex ratio imbalance for those below the poverty line is more striking than the overall figures. For instance, the sex ratio for those below the poverty level is 73:100, while the ratio drops to 69:100 among African Americans living in poverty (Aral, 1996). The effects of the sex ratio and employment on marital status are more evident under conditions of poverty (Taylor et al., 1997). Therefore, the belief that black men are in short supply is not a myth.

Secord and Ghee (1986) and Guttentag and Secord (1983) argued that sex ratio imbalance destabilizes existing relationships, because viable alternative mates are always available to the gender in short supply. The shortage of males leads to a context within which women tolerate male promiscuity and place themselves at risk for sexually transmitted infections by opting not to use condoms. In not using condoms, they are preserving the image of a relationship while trying to achieve long-term economic security and elevated social status.

Because of the scarcity of men and the importance of being attached to a man, women do not readily end relationships. Thus, they are willing to forgo protective behaviors such as condom use. In other words, women want to maintain the relationship even if it means risking HIV infection.

Baby's Mother
Another factor that affects condom use is a woman's position as baby's mother. Some women do not use condoms because they want a child by a particular man. They hope that this will result in a lifelong connection with the man. LaQuita explained why some women get pregnant.

> Some girls so much in love I want a baby by this boy. Or problems in their relationship and this gonna get pregnant by him and it's gonna bring us closer together. It's not gonna do that because I've done that. It's not gonna bring you no closer together.
>
> Younger people are confused because they think if you get pregnant by that boy you got a hold on him. You got that child and he gonna do for you and that child. That's what they figure. When they break up they get pregnant by this [another] guy. He gonna take care of me and my child. Then it's another guy. He's gonna take care of us now. It's all about money. They gonna do this for me. Buy me this. Do my nails, my hair. He gonna do. Next. Somebody will do it.
>
> All they figure is I got a baby. Yeah, you got a baby, but if you don't have help, it's rough. You gonna get stressed out, 'cause I got stressed out. (LaQuita)

Anna explained it this way:

> They are not called girlfriends. Your girlfriend is someone else, a completely different person. Everybody's got one. Everybody has a baby's mother. They have no plans to marry these people but they will do everything they can to be nice to them so they won't file child support.

For women, having a baby can be used to bond with a man and establish structural and economic links with the baby's father. While Worth (1989) found that women considered fathers simply "breeders" with no responsibility toward the child or woman, in the current study babies' mothers perceived financial responsibility from the father and an ongoing relationship with him. In reality, however, gaining financial responsibility from the baby's father and having an ongoing relationship with him is difficult or not realized. But baby's mother is still a socially prestigious position.

Baby's mother may or may not date other men. Shontele said:

> You're sort of like property then. The father can always go back and sleep with the baby's mother. It's like a given. He'll say I'll give you money. She'll say if you give me money I won't file child support. It's sort of like an intricate bartering system.

Yvonne explained that being baby's mother does not mean that you have the only connection to the father.

> Your girlfriend is someone else. Baby's mother is a good position to be in....You don't have sex with a lot of people. You become property. Father can always sleep with baby's mother. Fathers can sleep with anyone. You're like on the sidelines. But like a high level on the sidelines.

Being in a male/female relationship and having children elevates a woman's social status within the black community. Being baby's mother allows the mother to gain the status of womanhood if she is very young or still living with her parents. She also becomes an adult and can publicly maintain an ongoing relationship with the father. In this way the woman acquires social status and economic assistance (Hutchinson, 1999).

Women said they wanted to have a child to become a mother and have a family (43%), while others said they wanted "to have a part of themselves" (20%) or they "like kids" (11%). Women in this sample overwhelmingly want children (70%), but 58% do not have children and 61% believe you must be in a relationship to have a child. This creates a dilemma for this sample of lower-income women. On the one hand there is a desire for children and a relationship, but on the other is the perception that black men are in short supply (64%). Because of this gender imbalance women are more likely to be submissive to men (90%) and to put themselves at risk for STIs to maintain a relationship. This is suggested by women's involvement in the condom use decision-making process, where 73% stated that they made the decision together with their partner but 42% never use condoms, another 17% used condoms half the time or less, and 52% did not use a condom the last time they had sex. Women know the risk they are taking, because 66% believe it is very likely that they will get HIV if they do not use a condom. However, it is clear from the qualitative study and descriptive statistics that women do not believe that a condom should be used with a husband or boyfriend, even if he is unfaithful. In this sample of low-income black women, the desire for children and the security and social status of a male/female relationship outweighed the risk of sexually transmitted diseases such as HIV.

Pregnancy and Contraception
As reported in other studies (Worth, 1989), women do not think about getting pregnant until after sex. For instance, Yvonne noted:

> Guys don't want to hear anything about getting pregnant. If the girl gets pregnant, then she has to tell them. But that's like two months later and it's too late.

Other women in the intensive interviews were not concerned about pregnancy because they were in a relationship. They often said "if it happens, it happens." In other words, if they get pregnant, then it is meant to be.

Type of contraceptive used can be used to identify high- versus low-frequency condom users. Among the women in the intensive interviews, Yvonne periodically used the Pill, Latasha used Depo-Provera shots, Anna used condoms, and the other two women, LaQuita and Shontele, did not use any form of contraception, including condoms. In the survey, those who used condoms as their main form of contraception were more likely to be frequent condom users. In the survey, among those who used condoms as their main form of contraception, 30% used condoms more than half the time compared with 17% less than half the time. Among those who used other forms of contraception (such as the Pill) 42% used condoms half the time or less, compared with 11% using them more than half the time. Other studies indicate that use of oral contraceptives is related to decreased condom use among women (Kost & Forrest, 1992; Harvey, Beckman, & Wright, 1996; Lear, 1995; Upchurch et al., 1992). These women focused on the prevention of pregnancy rather than STI prevention (Detzer et al., 1995). In addition, switching from condom use to the Pill within a perceived stable relationship may symbolize serious commitment (Holland et al., 1990) and monogamy.

HIV and HIV Testing
The vast majority (92%) of the survey participants had been tested for HIV. Many were tested because they had had sex with someone without a condom (43%). For example, one woman was tested because she was "concerned about someone I had sex with," and another said she was tested because her cousin has AIDS. Others were tested during a routine physical exam (24%),

because of a pregnancy (11%), or blood exchange (8%). Their sexual partners were also tested (84%).

Guys in Yvonne's crowd did not discuss sexually transmitted diseases except in a joking way.

> We wouldn't talk about it. We would laugh about it but we wouldn't talk about it. There's this one scene in *Menace II Society*. This guy is on crack and he tells this dealer, "Man I'll suck your dick," and he ends up shooting him. In reality that's very, very true. They would talk about the guys who were on drugs. Man, you on crack, you probably got AIDS, and they'd laugh about it like that.

In the past, Latasha had gonorrhea. She is continually tested for HIV.

> I just felt like I need to be tested every six months. I said, every six months I'm going to take an HIV test. It's stressful because you go every six months and it's like I'm negative this six months but what about the next six months. It's horrible waiting on the results. It's stress on my mind. So you try to live every day like it's the last day of your life. You worry.

Latasha does not know if her boyfriend has been tested. She said "he's been in the hospital and they usually do that anyway." An HIV test does not challenge monogamy because it is justified as a routine medical procedure (Sobo, 1993).

Latasha discussed HIV with her partner, but "not the hard-core facts of it. We just let each other know that we don't want to deal with that. I'm just taking a risk that when he's with me he's with me and that it's just not going to happen."

LaQuita and her boyfriend had not been tested for HIV infection. When I asked why, she said, "It's love." In other words, maintaining the relationship is more important than HIV. She hopes that neither of them is infected, but whether or not she or he is HIV-seropositive, she wants to have unprotected sex with him. That is what it means to be in a relationship: unconditional sex. According to Detzer and associates (1995), low perceived need to use condoms is not related to low STI risk and actual STI risk is not related to condom use. Reasons for worrying about HIV/AIDS are related to infidelity and not the risk of infection. In other words, perceived risks for STIs, such as HIV, indicate a non-monogamous relationship. It is the lack of a committed relationship that concerns women, not the risk of HIV infection. Suggesting that a partner use a condom is similar to accusing him of being HIV infected (Moore & Rosenthal, 1991; Pivnick, 1993).

Two of the interviewees could distinguish between HIV and AIDS and knew how HIV was transmitted. For instance, Anna said:

> HIV is the virus that causes AIDS. AIDS is a killer. Acquired immune deficiency syndrome means immune system is screwed up....Get it from sex, needles, tainted blood.

Latasha also distinguished between HIV and AIDS.

> HIV is a deficiency. It's something that's in your system that your body doesn't have the ability to fight off. It's something that doesn't belong in your blood...AIDS is a terminal illness. HIV is a virus. AIDS is the full-blown disease. The end is coming. It's like a pneumonia.

Latasha believes people do not use condoms because they do not think they will get HIV/AIDS. She said:

> A lot of people feel, I can't get that. I won't get that. When I was younger I thought only homosexuals got it. When I lost my virginity I didn't use protection, but after that I always used protection. It scared me seeing the AIDS, gonorrhea, and syphilis. I think it's becoming more realistic because we had a lot of people die like Eazy-E. It's beginning to be reality. They need to know someone with it.

The other intensive interviewees thought HIV and AIDS meant the same thing. For instance, Yvonne said, "HIV and AIDS are the same things. People use the term AIDS...thought AIDS was a disease that drug addicts and gay people got...get AIDS from homosexual acts. White people, gay people, or people who do drugs." No one discussed perinatal transmission.

The image of sex as dangerous has been changed due to antibiotics, the Pill, and abortions (Holland et al., 1990). Individuals still think that medical technology can cure them, and that AIDS is a gay white male disease, although it is known that there is a disproportionately high prevalence among African Americans. For instance, LaQuita said:

> I grew up at a time when it [AIDS] was thought of as a gay white male disease. All you had to worry about was getting pregnant. I went to a predominantly white high school where white girls got pregnant and got abortions. So everything could be fixed. You know, if you've got a disease, it could be fixed. You just go down to the clinic and get a shot.

Shontele had her own ideas about the origin of the virus.

> Originated from wild sex with animals. A sheep or something. Things you not supposed to have sex with. Sex out of boundaries. People like having sex with animals, with things not supposed to be having sex with, just other living things. Gay men having sex with each other and gay women having sex with each other and gay men having sex with gay women and mixture of sex out of boundaries. Sex is where AIDS originated from.

While Shontele is aware that HIV and other STIs can be transmitted through heterosexual sex, she believes that "sex out of boundaries" is a more prevalent route of transmission.

One of the interviewees, Anna, stated that she was not worried about contracting HIV because she is more concerned about dying from daily living.

> I worry about dying crossing the street and trying to get into my car. I think more about the aspects of not dying from a disease as somebody trying to take my life from me, not necessarily dying from AIDS. I don't think about dying from AIDS.

Seventy-six percent of the survey respondents believe it is very likely that they will get HIV if they do not use a condom, but half did not use a condom the last time they had sex (52%). Risk of HIV infection is only one risk among many faced by black people in America.

While Anna and her partners discussed condoms, they did not discuss HIV. She does not feel the need to discuss HIV with her secondary partner, since they always use a condom, and she has not discussed HIV with her primary partner because "we haven't gotten to that point." This situation may be due to the need to feel that she is able to judge men. That is, to use a condom might mean that she is unintelligent and cannot determine a good man from a bad one. Using condoms also suggests that the man, or she herself, is diseased and not worth being a sex partner or long-term mate (Sobo, 1993).

DISCUSSION

According to gender role theory, gender stereotypes are culturally shared expectations for gender-suitable behaviors (Eagly, 1987). Gender identity is dependent on learning and social reinforcement that is reflected in gender-role behavior (feminine or masculine). Femininity in U.S. society socializes women to be passive sexually, to be pleasing to the dominant group, and in other ways (Amaro, 1995). In other words, to be feminine, women are socialized to be dependent, to lack initiative, and to be submissive and passive (Amaro, 1995; Miller, 1986). Such expectations encourage males and females to behave according to appropriate gender roles even during sexual interactions (Sacco et al., 1993). Consequently, women and men enter sexual relations with differing attitudes, behaviors, and expectations concerning condom use.

In addition, a woman's sense of self is based on the motivation to increase relationships with others. Maintenance of relationships has great meaning for women because of their basic orientation to others. Since women are subordinates, there is denial of their own needs; rather, they serve children, men, and family (Miller, 1986). "For many women the threat of disruption of *connections* [my italics] is perceived not just as a loss of a relationship but as something closer to total loss of self" (Miller, 1986, 83). Safer sex may be incompatible with the maintenance of these connections. That is, femininity is constructed in terms of connecting to others: males, children, and family. Therefore, cultural constructions of sexuality condition perceptions of risky sexual practices (Sobo, 1993).

Examination of the current sample of black women suggests that women cannot gain emotional fulfillment, economic security, and social status without a heterosexual relationship. However, they lack power in inter-gender sexuality. For poor women this lack of power within inter-gender relations is reinforced by the paucity of options for material survival outside of these relationships. In addition, more women than men practice monogamy and, for women, the affective relational context of sexual relations is important. That is, women prefer sexual relations based on intimacy, open communication, and mutual fidelity (Giffin, 1998). Condom use interferes with these goals.

In understanding the construction of condom use, we may take factors for granted that are not directly related to condoms. Women have more important issues to consider than sexually transmitted infections. They are concerned with economic survival, keeping the one they love, and having a family. In addition, because of the status acquired through a relationship with men and the importance of male attachments for black female identity, women may be willing to forgo protective behaviors such as condom use. This scenario occurs in a context of gender imbalance within a low-income environment. The outcome is to tolerate behaviors that one would not usually tolerate if there were a balance of power in inter-gender relationships. According to Sobo (1993, 466), "While sexual urges, a need to feel loved, the thirst for revenge, hunger for a child, or financial necessity can drive people to practice unsafe sex, sensed disempowerment facilitates it too."

Inconsistent condom use is linked to the meaning of female identity among African-American women. African-American women's cultural norms, including perceptions of black female identity, may place protective behaviors second to those ensuring the continuation of a relationship with a male partner. Americans, including African Americans, place high value on family and children. A relationship with male partners is one way to achieve this goal. Simultaneously, women may not have the educational background and skills to insure economic survival without assistance from a male partner. Consequently, the meaning of condom use is related to female identity and gender-role imbalance in an environment in which young black women live near or below the poverty level.

Notes

[1] Yvonne no longer frequents Nightclub X and has become an HIV/AIDS activist and social worker. She married the DJ at the club and they have a child. He decided to risk HIV infection not only to have a child, but "to have a normal relationship" with Yvonne. However, about three years after their child was born, her husband decided he could not handle living with someone with HIV, and they got a divorce. She continues to date but does not become intimate until she is ready to reveal her HIV status.

Bibliography

Amaro, H. (1995). Love, sex and power: Considering women's realities in HIV prevention. *American Psychologist, 50*(6): 437–447.

Amirkhanian, Y. A., Kelly, J., & Kabakchieva, E. (2003). Evaluation of social network HIV prevention intervention program for young men who have sex with men in Russia and Bulgaria. *AIDS Education and Prevention, 15*(3): 205–220.

Ananth, P., & Koopman, C. (2003). HIV/AIDS knowledge, beliefs, and behavior among women of childbearing age in India. *AIDS Education and Prevention, 15*(6): 529–546.

Aral, S. O. (1996). The social context of syphilis persistence in the southeastern United States. *Sexually Transmitted Diseases, 23*(1): 9–15.

Camlin, C. S., & Chimbwete, C. E. (2003). Does knowing someone with AIDS affect condom use? An analysis from South Africa. *AIDS Education and Prevention, 15*(3): 231–244.

Catania, J. A., Coates, T. J., Golden, E. G., Dolcini, M. M., Peterson, J., Kegeles, S., Siegel, D., & Fullilove, M. T. (1994). Correlates of condom use among black, Hispanic, and white heterosexuals in San Francisco: The AMEN longitudinal survey. *AIDS Education and Prevention, 26*(1): 12–26.

Catania, J. A., Coates, T. J., Stall, R., Turner, H., Peterson, J., Hearst, N., Dolcini, M. M., Hudes, E., Gagnon, J., Wiley, J., & Groves, R. (1992). Prevalence of AIDS-related risk factors and condom use in the United States. *Science,* 258: 1101–1106.

Cummings, G. L., Battle, R., Barker, J., & Krasnovsky, F. (1997). HIV risk among low-income African American mothers of elementary school children. *Journal of Health and Social Policy, 8*(3): 27–39.

Darity, W., & Myers, S. (1987). Public policy trends and the fate of the black family. *Humboldt Journal of Social Relations,* 14: 134–164.

Detzer, M., Wendt, S. J., Solomon, L. J., Dorsch, E., Geller, B. M., Friedman, J., Hauser, H., Flynn, B. S., & Dorwaldt, A. L. (1995). Barriers to condom use among women attending Planned Parenthood clinics. *Women and Health, 23*(1): 91–102.

Eagly, A. H. (1987). *Sex differences in social behavior: A social-role interpretation.* Hillsdale, NJ: Lawrence Erlbaum.

Ellerbrock, T., Bush, T. J., Chamberland, M. E., & Oxtoby, M. J. (1991). Epidemiology of women with AIDS in the United States, 1981 through 1990. *Journal of the American Medical Association, 265*(22): 2971–2975.

Flaskerud, J. H., & Nyamthi, A. M. (1989). Black and Latina women's AIDS related knowledge, attitudes, and practices. *Research in Nursing and Health,* 12: 339–346.

Flaskerud, J. H., & Rush, C. E. (1989). AIDS and traditional health beliefs and practices of black women. *Nursing Research, 38*(4): 210–215.

Fullilove, M. T., Fullilove, R. E., Haynes, K., & Gross, S. (1990a). Black women and AIDS prevention: A view towards understanding the gender rules. *The Journal of Sex Research, 27*(1): 47–64.

———. (1990b) Risk of sexually transmitted disease among black adolescent crack users in Oakland and San Francisco, California. *Journal of the American Medical Association,* 263: 851–855.

Geary, C. W., Tchupo, J. P., & Johnson, L. (2003). Respondent perspectives on self-report measures of condom use. *AIDS Education and Prevention, 15*(6): 499–515.

Giffin, K. (1998). Beyond empowerment: Heterosexualities and the prevention of AIDS. *Social Science and Medicine, 46*(2): 151–156.

Grinstead, O. A., Faigeles, B., Binson, D., & Eversley, R. I. (1993). Sexual risk for human immunodeficiency virus infection among women in high-risk cities. *Family Planning Perspective, 25*(6): 252–256, 277.

Gupta, G. R., & Weiss, E. (1993). Women's lives and sex: Implications for AIDS prevention. *Culture, Medicine and Psychiatry,* 17: 399–412.

Gupta, N., & Mahy, M. (2001). Sexual initiation among adolescent women and men: Trends and differentials in sub-Saharan Africa. Calverton, MD: Macro International, Demographic and Health Research Division.

Guttentag, M., & Secord, P. F. (1983). *Too many women: The sex ratio question.* Beverly Hills, CA: Sage.

Harvey, S. M., Beckman, L. J., & Wright, C. (1996). Perceptions and use of the male condom among African American university students. *International Quarterly of Community Health Education, 16*(2): 139–153.

Heise, L., & Elias, C. (1995). Transforming AIDS prevention to meet women's needs: A focus on developing countries. *Social Science and Medicine,* 40: 931–943.

Hinkle, Y.A., Johnson, E. H., Gilbert, D., Jackson, L., & Lollis, C. M. (1992). African-American women who always use condoms: Attitudes, knowledge about AIDS, and sexual behavior. *Journal of the American Medical Women's Association, 47*(6): 230–237.

Holland, J., Ramazanoglu, C., Scott, S., Sharpe, S., & Thomson, R. (1990). Sex, gender, and power: Young women's sexuality in the shadow of AIDS. *Sociology of Health and Illness, 12*(3): 336–350.

———. (1992). Risk, power, and possibility of pleasure: Young women and safer sex. *AIDS Care, 4*(3): 273–283.

Houston, L. N. (1981). Romanticism and eroticism among black and white college students. *Adolescence,* 16: 263–272.

Hutchinson, J. (1999). Hip hop generation: African American male-female relationships in a nightclub setting. *Journal of Black Studies, 30*(1): 62–84.

Jemmott, L. S., & Jemmott, J. B. (1991). Applying the theory of reasoned action to AIDS risk behavior: Condom use among black women. *Nurse Research,* 40: 228–234.

Johnson, E. H., Hinkle, Y., Gilbert, D., & Gant, L. M. (1992). Black males who always use condoms: Their attitudes, knowledge about AIDS, and sexual behavior. *Journal of the National Medical Association, 84*(4): 341–352.

Kline, A., Kline, E., & Oken, E. (1992). Minority women and sexual choice in the age of AIDS. *Social Science and Medicine, 34*(4): 447–457.

Kost, K., & Forrest, J. D. (1992). American women's sexual behavior and exposure to risk of sexually transmitted diseases. *Family Planning Perspectives, 24*(6): 244–254.

Ku, L., Sonenstein, F. L., & Pleck, J. H. (1994). The dynamics of young men's condom use during and across relationships. *Family Planning Perspective, 26*(2): 246–251.

Lear, D. (1995). Sexual communication in the age of AIDS: The construction of risk and trust among young adults. *Social Science and Medicine, 41*(9): 1311–1323.

Leigh, B. C. (1989). Reasons for having and avoiding sex: Gender, sexual orientation, and relationship to sexual behavior. *The Journal of Sex Research, 26*(2): 199–209.

Leigh, B. C., Temple, M. T., & Trocki, K. F. (1993). The sexual behavior of U.S. adults: Results from a national survey. *American Journal of Public Health,* 83: 1400–1408.

Leonard, D. (1980). *Sex and generation: A study of courtship and weddings.* London: Tavistock.

Lollis, C. M., Johnson, E. H., Antoni, M. H., & Hinkle, Y. (1996). Characteristics of African-Americans with multiple risk factors associated with HIV/AIDS. *Journal of Behavioral Medicine, 19*(1): 55–71.

Mays, V. M., & Cochran, S. D. (1988). Issues in the perception of AIDS risk and risk reduction activities by African-American and Hispanic/Latina women. *American Psychologist,* 43: 949–957.

Miller, J. B. (1986). *Toward a new psychology of women.* Boston: Beacon Press.

Moore, S. M., & Rosenthal, D. A. (1991). Condoms and coitus: Adolescents' attitudes to AIDS and safe sex behavior. *Journal of Adolescence,* 14: 211–227.

O'Leary, A., Goodhart, F., Jemmott, L. S., & Boccher-Lattimore, D. (1992). Predictors of safer sex on the college campus: A social cognitive theory analysis. *Journal of American College Health,* 40: 254–263.

Padian, N. S., Shiboski, S. C., & Jewell, N. P. (1991). Female-to-female transmission of human immunodeficiency virus. *Journal of the American Medical Association,* 266: 1664–1667.

Pivnick, A. (1993). HIV infection and the meaning of condoms. *Culture, Medicine and Psychiatry,* 17: 431–453.

Pleck, J. H., Sonenstein, F. L., & Ku, L. C. (1990). Contraceptive attitudes and intention to use condoms in sexually experienced and inexperienced adolescent males. *Journal of Family Issues, 11*(3): 294–312.

Radcliffe, K. W., Tasker, T., Evans, B. A., Bispham, A., & Snelling, M. (1993). A comparison of sexual behavior and risk behavior for HIV infection between women in three clinical settings. *Genitourinary Medicine,* 69: 441–445.

Reinisch, J. M., Sanders, S. A., Hill, C. A., & Ziemba-Davis, M. (1992). High-risk sexual behavior among heterosexual undergraduates at a midwestern university. *Family Planning Perspectives, 24*(3):116–121.

Richens, J., Imrie, J, & Copas, A. (2000). Condoms and seat belts: The parallels and the lessons. *Lancet, 355*(9201): 400–403.

Russell, K.Y., Wilson, M., & Hall, R. E. (1993). *Color complex: The politics of skin color among African-Americans.* New York: Harcourt Brace Jovanovich, Inc.

Sacco, W. P., Rickman, R. L., Thompson, K., Levine, B., & Reed, D. L. (1993). Gender differences in AIDS-relevant condom attitudes and condom use. *AIDS Education and Prevention, 5*(4): 311–326.

Sawyer, R., & Moss, D. (1993). Sexually transmitted diseases in college men: A preliminary clinical investigation. *Journal of American College Health,* 42: 111–115.

Secord, P., & Ghee, K. (1986). Implications of the black marriage market for marital conflict. *Journal of Family Issues, 7*(1): 21–30.

Selwyn, P., Hartel, D., Wasserman, W., & Drucker, E. (1989). Impact of the AIDS epidemic on morbidity and mortality among intravenous drug abusers in New York City methadone maintenance program. *American Journal of Public Health,* 79: 1360–1361.

Sobo, E. J. (1993). Inner-city women and AIDS: The psycho-social benefits of unsafe sex. *Culture, Medicine, and Psychiatry,* 17: 455–485.

———. (1995). Finance, romance, social support, and condom use among impoverished inner-city women. *Human Organization, 54*(2): 115–128.

Soet, J. E., Dilorio, C., & Dudley, W. N. (1998). Women's self-reported condom use: Intra and interpersonal factors. *Women and Health, 27*(4): 19–32.

Spradley, J. (1980). *Participant observation.* New York: Holt, Rinehart and Winston.

Svenson, G. R., Ostergren, P., & Merlo, J. (2002). Action control and situational risks in the prevention of HIV and STIs: Individual, dyadic, and social influences on consistent condom use in a university population. *AIDS Education and Prevention, 14*(6): 515–531.

Taylor, R. J., Tucker, M., Belinda, M., Chatters, L. M., & Bobakody, R. (1997). Recent demographic trends in African American family structure. In R. J. Taylor, J. S. Jackson, & L. M. Chatters (Eds.), *Family life in Black America* (pp. 14–62). Thousand Oaks, CA: Sage Publications.

Upchurch, D. M., Ray, P., Reichart, C., Celentano, D. D., Quinn, T., and Hook, E. W. (1992). Prevalence and patterns of condom use among patients attending a sexually transmitted disease clinic. *Sexually Transmitted Diseases, 19*(3): 175–180.

U.S. Department of Justice (1993). Bureau of Justice Statistics Special Report—HIV in U.S. Prisons and Jails. Bureau of Statistics.

White, J. L., & Parham, T. A. (1990). *The psychology of blacks: An African-American perspective.* Englewood Cliffs, NJ: Prentice Hall.

Wiggers, L. C. W., de Wit, J. R. F., & Gras, M. J. (2003). Risk behavior and social-cognitive determinants of condom use among ethnic minority communities in Amsterdam. *AIDS Education and Prevention, 15*(5): 430–447.

Wilson, W. J. (1987). *The truly disadvantaged: The inner city, the underclass, and public policy.* Chicago: University of Chicago Press.

Worth, D. (1989). Sexual decision-making and AIDS: Why condom promotion among vulnerable women is likely to fail. *Studies in Family Planning, 20*(6): 297–307.

Worth, D., & Rodriguez, R. (1987). Latina women and AIDS. *SIECUS Report, 15*(3): 5–7.

Wulfert, E., & Wan, C. K. (1993). Condom use: A self-efficacy model. *Health Psychology, 12*(5): 346–353.

CHAPTER THIRTEEN

Latex Condom Fashions

Thuy DaoJensen

At first glance, the work of Brazilian artist Adriana Bertini defies the tradition of conventional materials used to make works of art. Bertini creates imaginative women's clothing, from evening gowns to trendy two-piece outfits, out of latex condoms that have been dyed in brilliant colors, condoms that have been rejected by quality control persons within the condom industry.

Her interest in using latex condoms as "functional art" was inspired by her travels to social projects throughout Brazil. As a voluntary worker for GAPA (Grupo de Apoio a Prevencao de AIDS), an organization that provides support and helps in the prevention of AIDS, she became involved with promoting the message of safe sex practices through the use of condoms. When she received a box of 144 condoms that were past the expiration date, she developed an interest in condoms as a source of raw materials for her artistry. Since condoms are not biodegradable and the high levels of sulfur in burning condoms pollutes air quality, Bertini decided to create AIDS awareness through her works of "functional art" that allow the audience to contemplate the multifaceted ways in which the condom constitutes symbolic and practical issues and the risk of HIV throughout society. The question posed is: "How can we alert people of the danger of pleasure without advocating self-denial, which we know is impossible?"

The next few pages will offer a brief glimpse into Bertini's fanciful artwork of latex condoms in the form of women's clothing. Her web site informs us that "her work contains a pedagogical and informative character." In contrast to the controversial moralizing about promoting condoms as promoting promiscuity in the United States, Bertini's work provides a refreshing alternative in which art and aesthetics play a subtle yet powerful role in politicizing condom usage with fashion, environmental, and social issues.

Bibliography

Internet site: *www.adrianabertini.com.br*

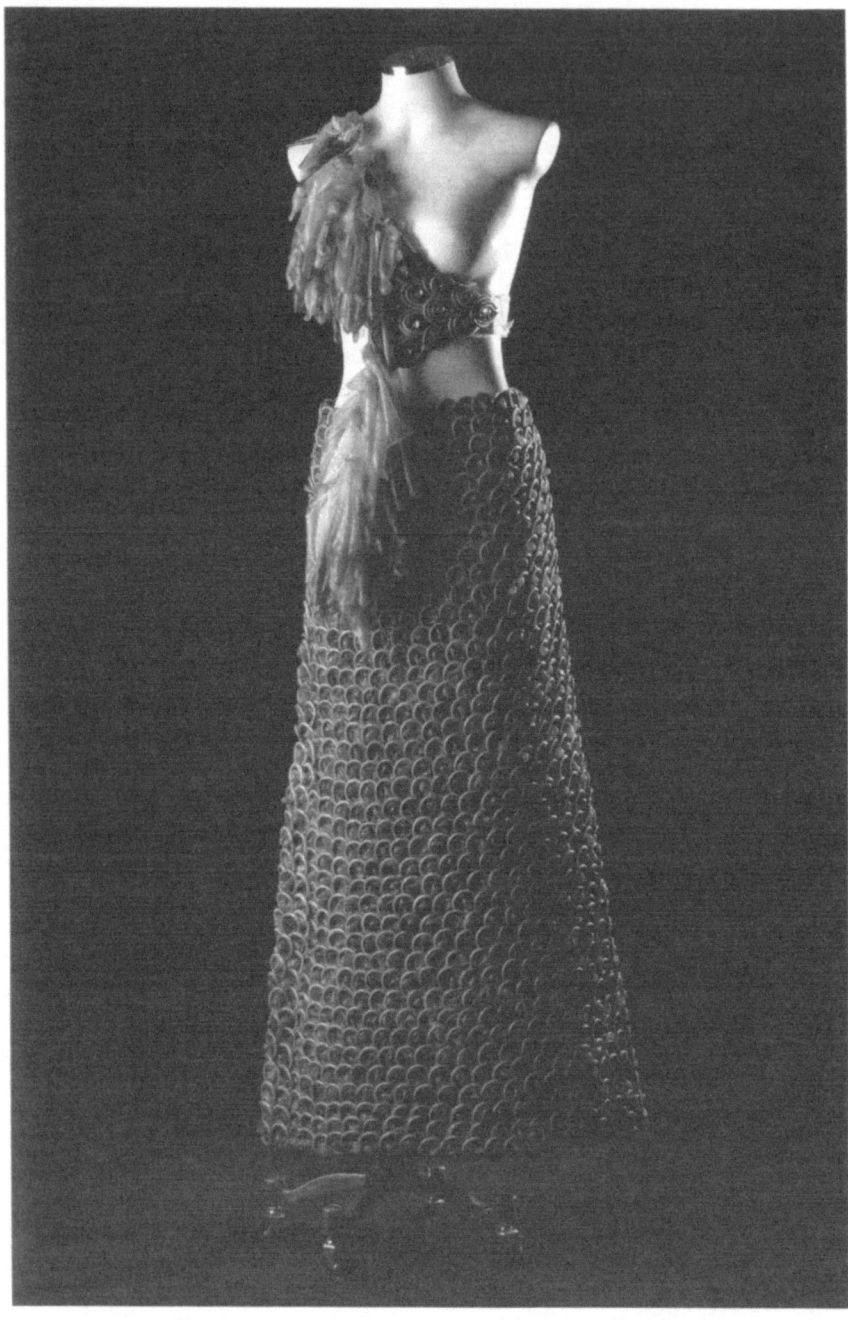

Dress Against the AIDS collection by Adriana Bertini (2003). Photography by Daniel Delaunay.

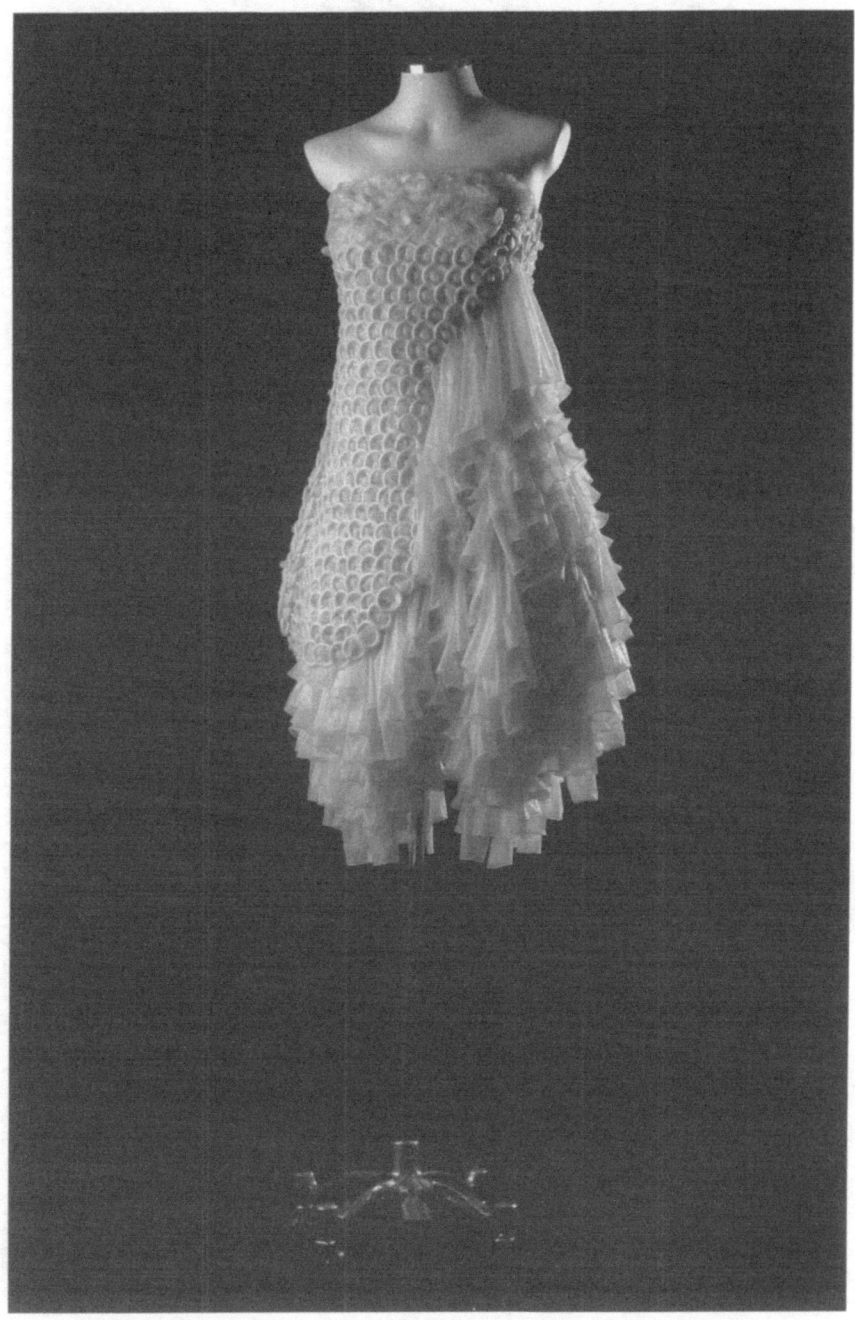

Dress Against the AIDS collection by Adriana Bertini (2003). Photography by Daniel Delaunay.

• Latex Condom Fashions •

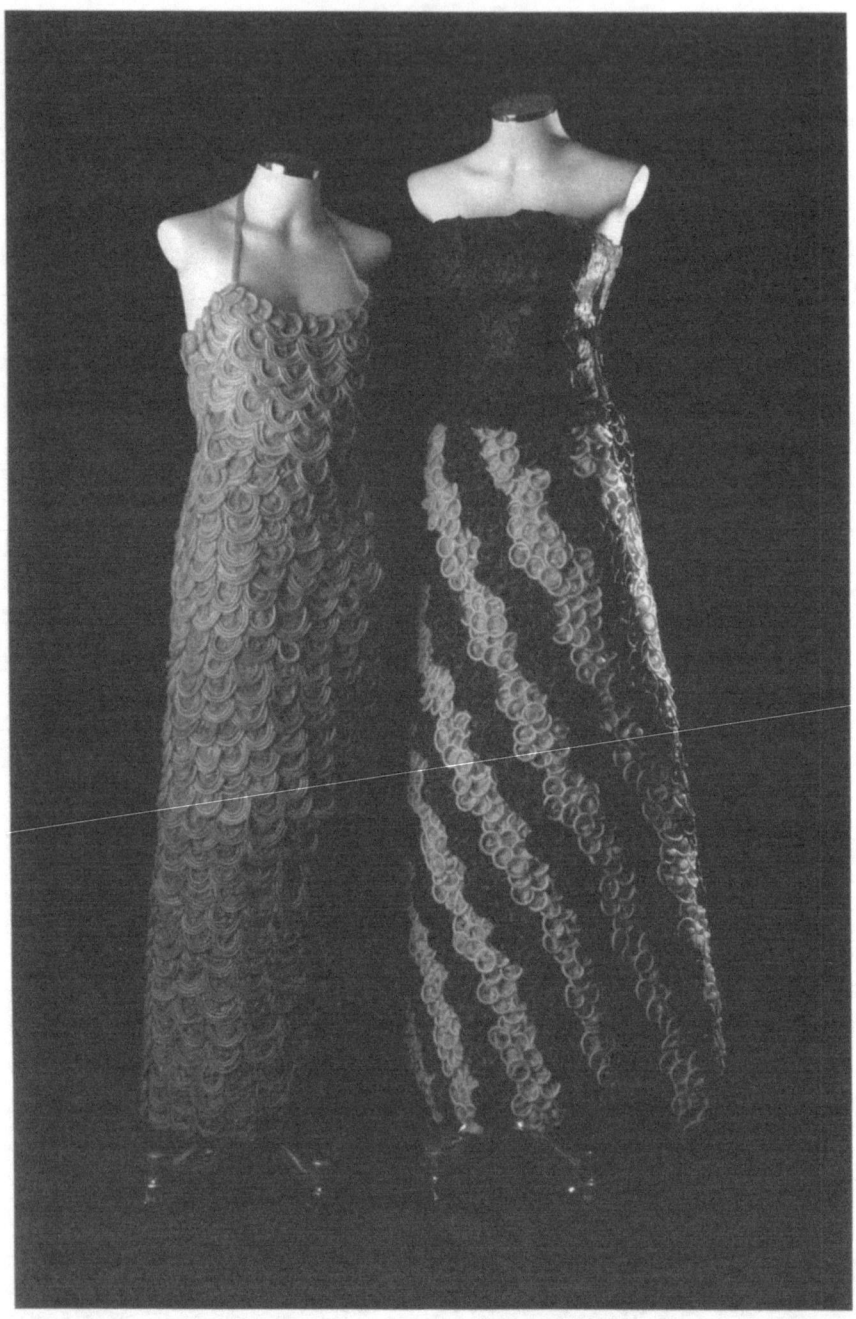

Dress Against the AIDS collection by Adriana Bertini (2003). Photography by Daniel Delaunay.

• Latex Condom Fashions • 167

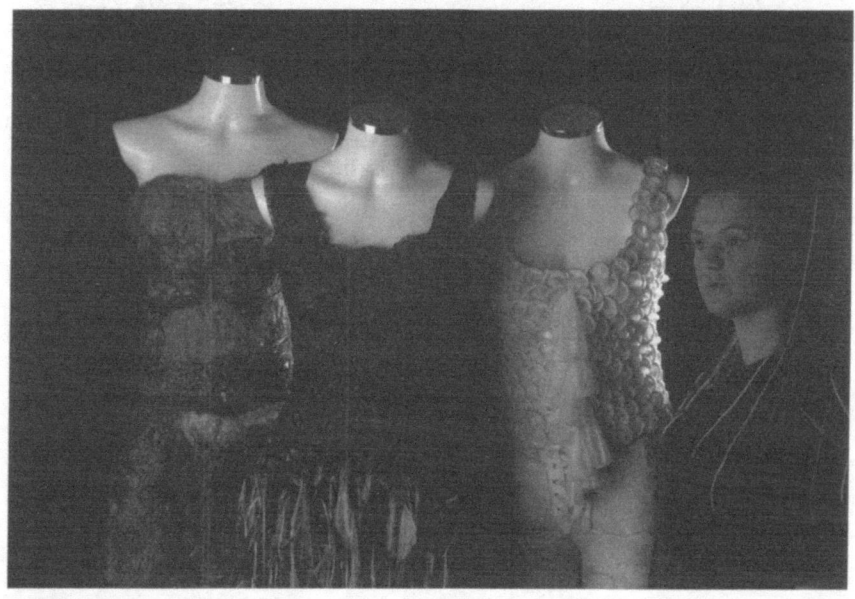

Dress Against the AIDS collection by Adriana Bertini (2003). Photography by Daniel Delaunay.

• Latex Condom Fashions •

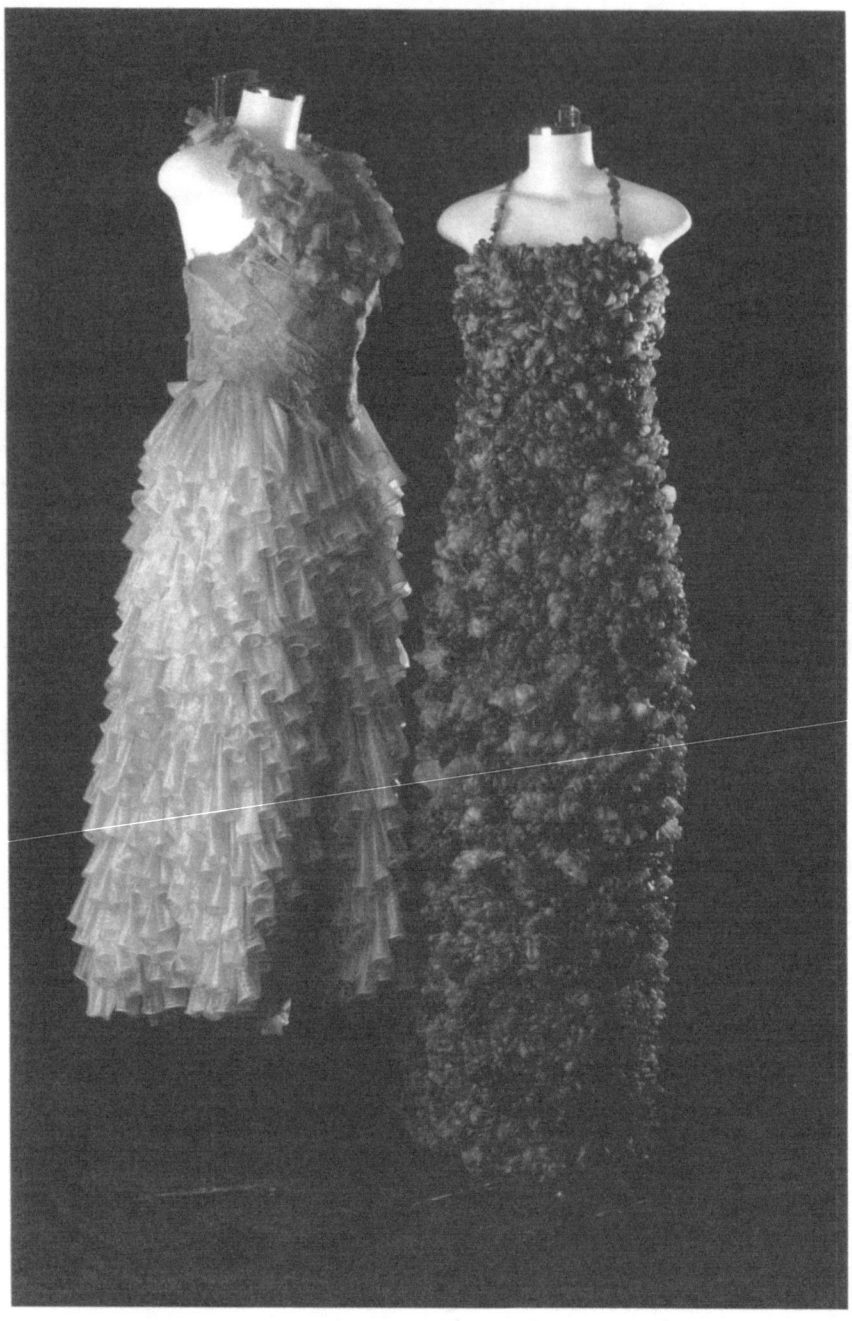

Dress Against the AIDS collection by Adriana Bertini (2003). Photography by Daniel Delaunay.

• CHAPTER FOURTEEN •

The Condom King

Vern L. Bullough

In Thailand, Mechai Viravaidya became so identified with the dissemination of condoms that his first name, Mechai, became synonymous with the condom. Called the Condom King by many of his admirers throughout the world, he is extremely proud of his self-identification with the condom in Thailand and still considers the popularization of the condom to be a major mission of his life, even as he has gone on to include other areas of economic and political development as well. His efforts to seek birth control for his fellow Thais—of which the condom became symbolic—have ranged from sponsoring contests blowing up condoms to the distribution of T-shirts with penises and condoms on them, from giving out king rings made of condoms to establishing a restaurant in Bangkok called Cabbages and Condoms, which is both a popular eating place and a condom museum. In the restaurant, condoms are everywhere. Trees in the courtyard are decorated with them; bouquets of flowers at each table are made from carefully rolled condoms; and condoms are displayed everywhere on the walls, ceiling, and floors, ranging in color, size, shape, and design, and made from a variety of materials. The attached museum and bookstore sells books and pamphlets about contraception and tourist souvenirs made of condoms. I should add that the meals served are of high quality. Though Mechai Viravaidya made his first mark in society as the Condom King, as of this writing he is a senator in Thailand's parliament

The son of two physicians who had met in Edinburgh while they were attending medical school, one of Scottish background, the other from Thailand, Mechai was born on January 17, 1941, the first son and second child of his parents. His name, Mechai, which literally means victory, was chosen by his parents to commemorate Thailand's then recent triumph in the French Indochina War. Each of the couple's four children was given a Thai name, and the parents worked hard to give their children a typical Thai childhood. In their early years all were sent to Thai schools. In the home, however, they learned English. Their mother usually spoke to them in English while the father spoke in Thai, but the children responded to both in Thai. At thirteen

Mechai was sent to an Anglican grammar school in Australia to, among other things, become more proficient in English. While in grammar school, he won a slogan-writing contest sponsored by a local radio station to publicize a dandruff remedy: "Of the wonders of the world, I have little notion. But the wonders of your hair is Page Barker's Scurf and Dandruff Lotion." His official biographer proclaimed that this success marked the birth of a "sloganeer."

Mechai made friends everywhere; in fact, he was so much of a social person that he generally ignored his studies. He had neither the ambition nor grades to get into a medical or law school, and instead went to a school of commerce. His extracurricular activities and lack of good study habits required him to spend five years instead of the more normal three years to complete his coursework. Though he could by no measure be classed as a high-achieving student, he remained well liked by his classmates and was a popular person on campus.

On his return to Thailand in 1965, the jobless Mechai fell into a position as escort on a national tour for the recently crowned Miss Universe, the first Thai woman to earn that honor. During the tour the press came to believe that he was romantically linked to the young woman (who already was in a committed relationship), and Mechai played to the press with the result that he, almost as much as she, became a national celebrity. When his stint as escort ended, the now "famous" Mechai, through the influence of his parents, was given a position at the National Economic Development Board assisting in the formulation of a five-year development plan. The position required him to travel extensively throughout Thailand, where the newspaper publicity of his association with the Miss Universe tour helped him meet people at all levels, not only those in government positions.

More or less unacquainted with Thailand as a country, he soon became aware through his travels of the wide scale of poverty and the large size of the families, something he vowed to himself to do something about. He was obviously ambitious also to become someone important. His first step on the path to bringing about change was to write a column, under a pseudonym, about issues of economic development for the *Bangkok World*, the English-language newspaper in Thailand read by many of the more influential people. Though he continued to write under a pseudonym, he made certain that an increasing number of the more influential Thais knew he was the author. This gave him greater influence in his agency and with the public than a newcomer could expect. He expanded his effort and, using another pseudonym, hosted a popular radio show in English and from there, finally abandoning the pseudonym, went on television and on stage.

In one of his pseudonymous newspaper articles, he had written a column about the lonely advocates of birth control in Thailand, and this led Allan Rosenfield, an official of the U.S.-based Population Council, to contact him. The result was a series of articles on population and family planning in the *Bangkok World* under Mechai's pseudonym but with data supplied by Rosenfield. The Ministry of Public Health, which already had taken a proactive approach to birth control, seized on the occasion to launch a Family Health Research Project in 1967 that concentrated on opening family planning centers in each district of the country. Mechai, while not directly involved in the program, was consulted and used his growing influence to push it. As he did so, he became increasingly frustrated with the government bureaucracy and felt he needed more power to have the program become more successful.

Ever politically aware, he decided the best way to push the program was to run for parliament. Unable to get an endorsement from a party in 1972, he ran as an independent. Though he lost, he had built an organization of supporters from whom he could draw in the future. After recovering from his defeat, the recently married Mechai (to Mom Ratchawongse Putrie Kritakara) took a part-time job as director of Information, Education, and Communication for the Planned Parenthood Association of Thailand. The Thai playboy had turned into a man with a mission. Although he had neither academic training nor specific experience with public relations and family planning, he did have important contacts in the media, was well known to the public at large, and had influential friends. He came to believe that the major problem facing Planned Parenthood was the need to overcome the societal reluctance to use contraceptives, something Mechai believed could be done through effective public relations campaigns.

The first step, he believed, was for people to feel comfortable with contraceptives and at ease with the topic of sex. He felt he needed a symbol that would both shock and titillate people. In looking at the available means of contraception then available in Thailand, the Pill, the IUD, and the condom, he decided to use the condom as a symbol in his public relations campaign, even though many Thais regarded pictorial representations of it as obscene. Though it was not mentioned, the widespread existence of American troops, either based in Thailand or there on R&R, meant that sexually transmitted diseases were also a major problem, and the condom was not only an effective contraceptive but could cut down the incidence of STDs as well.

Mechai believed that if he could get people to laugh about the condom, he could challenge the social proscriptions against contraceptives. He began by distributing condoms much as he would his personal name card at official functions and social occasions, but also at bus stations, in hotel lobbies, in front of movie theaters—in fact, anywhere people gathered and he was present. He also gave them in lieu of tips to parking lot attendants and others. He found that the first reaction was surprise, then shock, usually followed by laughter as the condom was being pocketed. Mechai then proceeded to the next step by producing stickers, posters, T-shirts with catchy slogans, and the staging of media events that drew the press. He seized on any item. When he heard that a foreign expatriate had a vasectomy at a Thai clinic, Mechai invited the press to publicize the event (but not the name of the individual) in order to demonstrate that since Thai clinics were good enough for Westerners, they should be good enough for Thais.

His campaign was not without hostile response, and one critic wrote that if he liked the condom so much, the condom should be called a "mechai" to see just how much he liked it. Mechai, ever the extrovert, seized on the new term simply to publicize the condom, even though it meant that he might forever be identified with it. There was considerable criticism of him and his self-publicity within the Planned Parenthood Association of Thailand. To counter the criticism, he stacked the annual membership meeting in 1973 with two busloads of members whom he had recruited, and they proceeded to vote him into the position of secretary general of the association.

One of his major efforts was to send his message to the local villages, and though he had initially arranged for volunteer physicians to prescribe oral contraceptives in a pilot project, he soon came to believe that this role in the village could best be filled by nonphysicians. The success of this new action was quickly demonstrated and it became the model for what he wanted to do. Mechai's brash self-publicizing methods proved increasingly irritating to the Thai official Planned Parenthood organization. As opposition to him mounted as his two-year term was coming to an end, he resigned rather than engage in what would have been a hotly contested election just as his village plans were about to begin.

His resignation cut him off from funds from the International Planned Parenthood Federation, because bylaws permitted only one group in a country to be the official group. In spite of this, the IPPF, believing in what he was trying to do, determined to support his village project even if it had to go outside its regular channels to do so. Mechai quickly formed a new organization, Community Based Family Planning Services, to extend his experimental plan to seventy-six communities in Thailand, Vietnam, Laos, and Cambodia, the Mekong Delta countries. Since the organization was regional and not national, funds could be given. In 1974, the IPPF gave a $250,000 one-year grant for this project, and Mechai and his staff were off and running their new NGO (Non-Governmental Organization). He developed solutions to all kinds of red tape barriers. For example, nonphysician distribution of contraceptives by anyone not of the Ministry of Public Health was then illegal in Thailand. Mechai, however, was able to get around this by labeling his new program as an experimental one, and the government was hesitant to move against him. He immediately began to get his distribution plan in action. In the initial experiment some twenty-four villages were chosen, volunteers were trained, and contraceptive information and devices began to be distributed. It soon became quite clear that if contraceptives were distributed by a local woman whom the village women knew and trusted, they did not hesitate to use them, even if they had to pay for them. The payment scheme he developed was simple. Each cycle of pills cost five baht (then about twenty-five cents U.S.), while five condoms cost three. The program allowed the village distributor to keep one baht of each sale as an incentive, with the remainder remitted to the project to defray costs of training and administration. A district supervisor visited each village distributor once a month to examine records, answer questions, resupply contraceptives, and collect funds. As soon as the experiment proved successful, Mechai was able to get the Thai government to change its policy as well. The IPPF continued to fund him as he expanded the program by offering a family planning course for teachers during the summer to upgrade their qualifications and skills.

Among other things, teachers were taught new rhymes and songs to be introduced into the classroom. Learning the English alphabet was tied in with the ABCs of birth control, with A for Abstinence, B for Birth spacing, C for Condoms, D for delayed marriage, S for sterilization, V for vasectomy, and so on. A popular Thai jingle was written in which words were changed in order somehow to have every contraceptive method mentioned. Demographic messages explaining the dangers of overpopulation were developed. To keep teachers interested, condoms were blown up and desensitization sessions were held so the teachers would feel comfortable. Mechai continued to practice what he preached, and when he was invited to attend a meeting of Vietnamese delegates to Thailand, he passed out condoms to each. The Vietnamese eventually adopted his program themselves.

Mechai's success was demonstrated by the rapid decline in the fertility rate, one of the most rapid ever recorded. By 1981, Thailand's total fertility rate had fallen to 3.9 from its peak of 7.4 in the 1960s. The population growth rate had plummeted from 3.33 percent in 1960 to 2 percent by 1980 and 1.6 percent by 1984. In more tangible terms, Thailand's population, which had been doubling every twenty-one years, would now do so only every forty-four years. Rates have continued to drop until by 2002 the total fertility rate was measured at 2, and some 70 percent of all women aged fifteen to forty-nine were using modern methods of contraception.

Obviously multiple factors were at work, including effective government policy planning, but the village councils remained the key. Mechai, ever the innovator, went further in an attempt to combine family planning with economic development. He began slowing adding to his program: Farmers using family planning could rent a team of buffalo to plow their fields at half price, or they could use the services of a Family Planning Stud Pig at special rates. Low-interest loans were given to people using family planning, and they could buy livestock and insecticides at a lower rate. Using its existing network, the Community Based Family Planning Services established a "Better Marketing Program," acting as a distributor so the families could sell directly to the market without going through a middleman. This program also helped the program become more economically self-sufficient. A Village Development Fund was established, which gave cash incentives to individuals who had vasectomies, female sterilization, used IUDs, injectable contraceptives, or pills. The program expanded to include cash to women who did not get pregnant in any single year, and in some cases, every month where no pregnancy was reported. Mechai also opened abortion clinics for those women who had an unwanted pregnancy. Abortion could not be performed, however, without counseling that the program encouraged both the man and woman involved to attend so that both could understand the ramification of the procedure. In each case, it was also emphasized that pregnancy was preventable if modern contraceptives were used properly.

As his organization grew and expanded, Mechai felt that he needed an umbrella organization to oversee the growing variety of projects. In 1976, he established the Population and Community Development Association (PDA). His old agency, the CBFPS, was one agency within PDA. In 1977, all profit-making activities from clinics to paraphernalia were subsumed under the title of the Population and Development Company (PDC), and it became a private for-profit company independent of PDA. By its charter, however, profits could be used only for charitable purposes.

As his reputation grew, Mechai continued to explore new fields, both in governmental and private posts. For a time he served as governor of the Provincial Water Works Authority, then as deputy minister of industry, a position from which he resigned to become a visiting scholar at Harvard in 1988. On his return, and again heading up the PDA, he became involved in the AIDS problem in Thailand. This was complicated by the Thai reputation for hospitality and a political combination of brothel owners and others in the sex industry, police, and politicians, all worried that a full-fledged campaign would weaken the tourist industry. Mechai again pushed the use of condoms but with less humor than before, because the issue was now a life-and-death struggle for the survival of Thailand. The television and radio stations in Thailand under various forms of government control initially had refused to broadcast his message about the AIDS epidemic, but finally he persuaded the army, which controlled 326 radio and 2 television stations, to join with him in mobilizing a national effort to combat AIDS. By 1991, Mechai had won his battle and was put in charge of developing a national plan for prevention of AIDS/HIV. Soon after this he was named minister of tourism, public information and mass communications by the new government that had come into power. Included in his portfolio was the coordination of the National AIDS Prevention and Control Program, which Mechai used to publicize the country's fight against AIDS.

Never one to stop exploring, Mechai renewed his interest in economic development in Thailand and, through his PDA organization, enticed a number of industries to establish plants in Thailand. At the same time, he continued public service as chair of the Board of the Telephone Organization of Thailand. In 1998, he became chair of the Board of the Krung Thai Bank, then Thailand's largest state-owned commercial bank, a position from which he resigned when his reforms were ignored. His next step was to campaign for and be elected to the Thai Senate, a position he holds as of this writing.

In 1997, he received the United National Population Award for his "outstanding contribution to the awareness of population questions and to their solutions." He still prides himself on the title of Condom King, and his restaurant, Condoms and Cabbages, continued to be an important tourist spot in Bangkok. No one has yet been able to match his ability to publicize and popularize condoms.

Bibliography

Bullough, V. (2001). *Encyclopedia of birth control.* Santa Barbara, CA: ABC-CLIO.

d'Agnes, T. (2001). *From condoms to cabbages: An authorized biography of Mechai Viravaidya.* Bangkok, Thailand: Post Publishing Company.

• CHAPTER FIFTEEN •

Family Planning and Male Friendships:
Sathi Condom and Same-Sex Sexual Desire
Among Men in Pakistan

Ahmed Afzal

On a late summer night, a lone dimly lit streetlight reveals silhouettes of two men sitting on the concrete steps of a nameless grocery store. Wearing the traditional shalwar kameez, a loose-fitting knee-length shirt and trousers, the two men are smoking cigarettes. It is hard to tell whether they are chatting or just silently watching the night pass by, comfortable in each other's company. The grocery store is located in a deserted section of a low-income neighborhood in Rawalpindi, a midsized city in the province of Punjab in Pakistan.[1] Across from the grocery store is an open field of patchy grass that is packed during the day with young boys playing cricket.

I walk toward the two men, Aamir and Sohail. I have known them for over three years and have developed close friendships with both. Most of the business for the day has already concluded by this time, and there are hardly any customers who come to the store in the late evening. On most days, I can find Sohail and Aamir sitting together on the front steps of Sohail's grocery store.

I met Aamir through a common friend some years back and we quickly became friends. Although Aamir had been involved in a sexual relationship with Sohail when we first met, it was several months before I actually met Sohail and learned that they were more than just platonic friends.

On this particularly humid late summer night, I am carrying with me a bag of Trojan condoms to give to Aamir and Sohail. As I approach the two, Aamir gets up, pulls me in a tight hug, and holds my hand. "Where have you been? We haven't seen you in several days. You have forgotten about us," he says in Urdu. "I was away for work and just returned yesterday," I say in the way of an explanation.

We chat about work, and Aamir and Sohail fill me in on the goings-on in their lives since I last saw them about a month ago.

Sohail notices the brown paper bag I am carrying and asks, "What's in the bag?"

I take out the Trojan condoms.

"Oh, you brought 'Sathi' for us," Aamir says somewhat casually.

"I got them for you," I tell him, noticing for the first time Aamir's renaming of Trojan condoms as Sathi.

"Yaar, I don't like Sathi. I can't come wearing Sathi....It is so tight," Aamir frowns, as he holds up the nonlubricated latex condom in red packaging.

"But you have to wear it," Sohail tells Aamir.

Aamir pulls Sohail toward him and holds him in a tight embrace. "What, are you worried you'll get pregnant? You know I don't like wearing Sathi. I'll use it when I get married," he says playfully. "I don't feel anything when I wear it...bilkul maza nahi aata (I feel absolutely no pleasure)...but I'll wear it for you."

Aamir and Sohail were among several men I met during the course of my research on the attitudes of Pakistani men toward sexual health and HIV/AIDS (Afzal, 1995). The research provided me with an opportunity to analytically examine cultural conceptions of male sexualities within the context of intimate friendships, and gendered public and private spaces of male sociality in Pakistan. In the course of this research from 1993 until 1997, I became close friends with several of these men, and as deeply involved in their lives as they became in mine.

All of these men were Punjabi, the dominant ethno-linguistic group in the province of Punjab in Pakistan. All of them resided in low-income localities in Rawalpindi. All men, like me, were Muslim,[2] single, in their early twenties, and lived in extended family households. Several were employed in the private sector. Others, like Aamir, worked in middle- to lower-tier positions in governmental agencies. Faisal was a full-time cab driver. Sohail owned his own grocery store. The youngest of my friends, Reza, had just recently completed high school and was working as a receptionist at a local hotel.

The commonality among these men extended beyond shared ethno-linguistic and class identities and affiliations, to the realm of sexuality: All of these single men were involved in romantic relationships with men. In spite of having sexual relationships with other men, none self-identified as "homosexual" or even "bisexual." Indeed, such definitions of a fixed sexual identity had very little meaning in their lives or spoke to their construction of a fluid, culturally informed male sexuality that permitted an eroticization of both women *and* men. A critical component of such a culturally constructed male sexuality is an absence of anxiety regarding sexual relationships with men.[3]

Indeed, sexual relationships between men like Aamir and Sohail were a natural progression in the individually negotiated terrain of intimate close friendships. As another friend, Ali, whom I also met during the course of my research, told me: "Well, I would never even think about being with any other man except my childhood friend. We had been friends for so long that it seemed only *natural* that we would eventually 'be together [sexually].' But I would never cross the line with someone I did not know as well, and feel as strongly for."

Within this group of single Punjabi men, sexual relationships with men were exemplified by clearly articulated active and passive sexual roles for both partners. The active sexual role is defined by the sexual act of penetration, and the passive role assumed by the partner who is penetrated. Anthropological studies of male sexuality in South American cultures (for example, Carrier, 1976; Lancaster, 1988; Parker, 1986 and 1999; Taylor, 1986) provide rich theoretical and ethnographic insights into constructions of sexuality premised on sexual roles—that is, active or passive—rather than sexual identity: homosexual, bisexual, or heterosexual.

Ethnographic research with Punjabi men like Sohail, Aamir, and Ali shows similar configurations of male sexual desire and relationships. In Pakistan, as in most South American cultures, the active partner's engagement in the sexual act poses no threat to his masculinity and manhood and his social identity as an adult and implicitly heterosexual male. Indeed, his ability to penetrate both women *and* men sexually contributes to an elevated status within his close circle of friends, privy to the sexual relationships with men. The passive partner, on the other hand, remains vulnerable to being undermined as a "real man," his masculinity and manhood sometimes in question. The act of being penetrated sexually—culturally conceived as feminine—contributes to a feminization of the passive male partner, at least in the realm of sexual contact and interaction. Not surprisingly, within such a cultural configuration of same-sex male desire, sexual relations between men become loosely modeled on established local patterns of male-female marital relationships.

Although most of these men appropriate established local patterns of heterosexual, male-female marital relationships in organizing same-sex sexual relationships, the organization of permissible sexual activities and behavior is a distinctly unique facet of same-sex eroticism. Sexual behavior and activities are individually negotiated and vary from couple to couple. Indeed, both male partners mutually establish and negotiate the boundaries of sexual play, including kissing, oral sex, and even penetration. Ali, for example, told me matter-of-factly that his boyfriend, Reza, was uncomfortable kissing on the lips or giving oral sex. On the other hand, Sohail shared with me that Aamir freely kissed him and performed oral sex, but always refused to be penetrated sexually. Rahim's repertoire of sexual activities was limited to caressing, kissing, and oral sex. "I cannot bear the idea of being penetrated. I think I am more passive, though, because I wouldn't want to penetrate my [male] partner either," Rahim told me during one of our more candid conversations at his home.

Despite such anxiety-free assertions of the naturalness of same-sex erotic desire, and individually negotiated sexual roles within such friendships, almost all men, including Ali and Reza, planned to eventually marry a woman and raise a family. At first, the desire for marriage and children might be seen as familial expectation. Yet most Punjabi men I met *wanted* to marry and raise a family. Over the course of my research, I realized that for these Punjabi men, marriage and children were integral to a sense of a masculine self and adulthood. A sexual relationship between men appeared to have its own valued place; intimate same-sex relationships did not replace, threaten, or marginalize heterosexual desire or relationships. It is within such broad contours of a culturally constructed male sexuality that one can begin to understand the everyday negotiations of same-sex sexual desire with the heteronormative ideals of family and marital life in Pakistan, the cornerstones of the Pakistani state policy on population control, family planning, and condom usage.

The interaction in front of the grocery store with which I begin this essay illustrates one of the contexts within which I formed friendships and interacted with men who had sex with men and elicited ethnographic data on their attitudes toward HIV/AIDS and issues of male sexuality. As discussed in the preceding section, the interaction is suggestive of cultural constructions of intimate male friendships.[4] Equally significant, the interaction also illuminates a specific discourse on condoms and male sexuality within gendered spaces of male sociality and interaction in contemporary urban Pakistan. I had brought with me a box of an American brand of latex condoms to give to Aamir and Sohail. Yet the primary interpretive framework for Aamir to speak of "condoms" was one that was informed by a locally marketed and distributed brand of condom called Sathi.

Sathi is the Urdu word for a companion or a friend. Aamir's "renaming" of the Trojan condoms, and indeed *all* condoms, as Sathi is part of a larger story of the conception, marketing, and distribution of the Sathi condom among low-income urban populations in Pakistan during the 1980s and 1990s. The story is also about the ways in which men like Aamir and Sohail enter this larger narrative about Sathi condoms through their creative appropriation of the heteronormative Pakistani state discourse and practices on family planning and marriage, and even nationhood.

This essay is an attempt to tell a version of this story. It is a version that accounts for the complex interactions among international, national, and local contexts and situations that led to the production and marketing of the Sathi condom in the mid-1980s in Pakistan. In telling this story, I highlight the intersection of varied interests—that of international development agencies, the Pakistan state bureaucracies, and the private sector—in the production of the Sathi condom. Specifically, Pakistan state agencies, in collaboration with international development agencies and Pakistani and American private sector organizations, had produced and marketed the Sathi condom specifically for heterosexual married couples from low-income groups in urban Pakistan.

The Sathi condom was marketed as the primary method of "responsible family planning" and intended by the Pakistan state to contribute to the construction of a modern Pakistani citizen. Indeed, the Pakistan state discourse on family planning and social and sexual reproduction privileged heterosexual married couples as the site for constructing modern Pakistani citizens. What is notable is that private national and international interests colluded with the Pakistan state to relegate a modern Pakistani citizenry and condom usage to the *exclusive* domain of heterosexual marriage and marital sex.

I argue that a segment of Pakistani men who have sex with men enter the story of the Sathi condom through their creative appropriation of the heteronormative ideology of the Pakistan state. By virtue of its name, *Sathi* or friend, the condom intersected the realm of culturally informed intimate and often sexual relationships between male friends in Pakistan in which men often refer to their close, intimate friend as their Sathi. Such epistemological expansion of the word indicates the possibility of men like Aamir and Sohail becoming situated within the state's project of constructing modern Pakistani citizens, while also making visible expressions of an alternative, non-heteronormative sexuality.

This creative appropriation of a decidedly heteronormative state ideology is significant because it enables the retelling of the story of the Sathi condom that accounts for the myriad contexts and expressions of male sexuality in contemporary Pakistan, and contests the construction of nation, male sexuality, and citizenship as essentially heterosexual. Moreover, the analysis has important implications for family planning and population control initiatives and policy, and for ethnographic studies of marriage and male sexuality. In telling this story, I locate the origins of Sathi condom in the Pakistan state discourse, programs, and practices on family planning and population control in the decades following the formation of Pakistan in 1947, the subject of the following section.

Genealogies of Sathi Condom:
Pakistan State, Family Planning, and the Regulation of Sexuality
The Sathi condom was launched in 1986, a period marked by the transnational circulation of ideologies of sustainable development. By the 1980s, rapid population growth had featured prominently on the policy agenda in Pakistan. Sustainable development, that is, the enhancement of peace, social justice, and well-being within and across generations, emerged as the panacea for the crisis of rapid population growth in Pakistan. With over 140 million inhabitants, Pakistan is the world's seventh most populous nation. According to United Nations projections, the population will grow to 285 million by 2050, at which time Pakistan will rank as the world's fourth most populous country (Sultan, Cleland, & Ali, 2002). The United Nations report attributes this enormous projected increase to a slow pace of fertility decline, in spite of little evidence to support that Pakistani married couples wanted particularly large families (Sultan et al., 2002). Yet most public initiatives to contain the population growth had "borne" minimal success (Cernada & Bob, 1992; Maudlin & Ross, 1994; Rosen & Conly, 1996; Sathar, 1993).

Containment of population growth, however, was not a late-twentieth-century public policy imperative in Pakistan. In fact, Pakistan was one of the first countries to develop a national population program in order to effectively control the rapid population growth. Eight years after independence from British colonial rule and the creation of an independent Islamic Republic of Pakistan, the Pakistan Population Program began in 1953 in the private sector and was operationalized through a voluntary association, the Family Planning Association of Pakistan. In its first five-year development plan (1955–1960), the government of Pakistan provided financial support for the Family Planning Association with the objective of "motivating couples and providing family planning services" (Ministry of Population Welfare, 2002). Subsequent five-year development plans similarly conceptualized population control through family planning as a prerequisite for a modern Pakistani subjectivity and citizenship. The state's conception of a modern Pakistani citizenship was located in the exclusive domain of marriage, and defined by smaller family size and spacing in births.

The state's intervention in the realization of such ideals of modern citizenship and subjectivity contributed to the creation of a federal government ministry. The Ministry of Health and Family Welfare, and since 1990, the Ministry of Population Welfare, functions as the central state institution responsible for all population-related policies and programs in Pakistan. The Ministry of Population Welfare's communication campaigns provide a lens for understanding how the state deems heterosexual marriage as the only publicly legitimated domain for sexual relations and constructs the small family as the site for conferring a modern Pakistani citizenship. Consider the mission statement for the Ministry of Population Welfare's communication campaigns. According to the ministry, its objectives include:

> increasing knowledge of population programs to create urgency to adopt and promote family planning measures for a small and prosperous, happy family; to minimize the predominance of son preference; to promote concept and practice of marriage at mature ages and promote spacing in child [births] for the health of the mother and children. (Information, Education, and Communication: Past Campaigns)

The mandate of the Ministry of Population Welfare goes further than merely increasing knowledge regarding the importance of smaller family size; it also includes the planning, development, monitoring, and evaluation of all publicly funded programs relating to the regulation and control of population growth in Pakistan. The Population Welfare Program is the cornerstone of the ministry's activities. According to the official ministry web site, the "mission" of the Population Welfare Program is defined as follows:

> The Population Welfare Program is an ongoing social development endeavor operating within the framework of nationally accepted, broad-based and strategically focused population and development policies. The mission of the Ministry centers on population issues with a view to achieve replacement level fertility for population stabilization. It emphasizes...the improvement and enrichment of the quality of life of individuals, families and communities within the framework of reproductive health, instead of pursuing demographic targets in isolation. (Mission Statement, the Ministry of Population Welfare)

In fulfilling this mandate, the Pakistan state utilized electronic and print media as crucial vehicles for the "communication and propagation of advantages and importance of small family norms" (Brief, Ministry of Population Welfare, Government of Pakistan).

The number of annual surveys carried out by the Pakistan state agencies to document the prevalence of contraceptive use is almost obsessive, and they attest to the state's persistence in regulating male and female sexuality. The National Fertility Survey, Pakistan Contraceptive Prevalence Survey, Family Planning Survey, and the Pakistan Demographic and Health Survey are just some of the main surveys carried out annually. These surveys target married women aged between fifteen and forty-nine and attempt to provide quantifiable data such as mean age at marriage, correlations between literacy level and fertility rates among married women, contraceptive prevalence rate, and family size.

The Pakistan state's preoccupation with "family planning" through documentation of contraceptive usage practices and behaviors reveals as much the crisis of population growth in Pakistan as it does the role of the state as a hypervigilante with a "mission" to control and regulate the familial and domestic space of the family, and by extension, nation through intervention in reproductive health. Ideologically framed phrases such as "family planning" and "small family norms" feature prominently in all literature of the Ministry of Population Welfare, and mark the family, community, and nation as essentially heterosexual. M. Jacqui Alexander's 1997 essay on the 1991 Sexual Offenses and Domestic Violence Act in the Bahamas suggests the universality of the production of the nation, family, and citizenship through a regulated heterosexual sexuality that is applicable to Pakistan:

> The nation has always been conceived in heterosexuality, since biology and reproduction are at the heart of its impulse. The citizenship machinery is also located here, in the sense that the prerequisites of good citizenship and loyalty to the nation are simultaneously sexualized and hierarchized into a class of good, loyal, reproducing heterosexual citizens, and a subordinated, marginalized class of non-citizens. (p. 471)

In her discussion of the existence of alternative sexualities within dominant nationalism, Gayatri Gopinath (1997) similarly argues that heterosexuality is fundamental to the way in which the nation imagines itself and all non-heteronormative subjects "are written out of national memory entirely" (1997: 469–70). Not surprisingly, Sathi condom was conceived within the paradigm of a heterosexual citizenship and situated within the exclusive domain of heterosexual and procreative marital sex.

However, this is not the complete story of the Pakistan state project. Male sexuality in Pakistan, as in certain other cultural and national contexts, particularly in South America, materializes through its complex interaction with larger cultural formations. For example, although several Pakistani men who have sex with men belie easy categorization as either homosexual or even bisexual, they are nonetheless able to situate themselves within the state's hegemonic construction of citizenship and nation. Men like Aamir, Sohail, and several others whom I interviewed did not reject marriage and "family planning" or position themselves outside of the state project of citizenship and nationhood, defined in heteronormative terms. However, through their valued intimate friendships with men, they reconfigured the hegemonic discourse to make visible their own construction of an alternative sexuality that coexists with local ideals of marriage, family life, and procreation.

In the following section, I examine the construction of an alternative sexuality by a segment of lower-middle-class men in urban Punjab, to illuminate the everyday contestations and reconfigurations of the dominant discourse on family planning premised on a *naturalized* association among marriage, martial sex, and modern citizenship.

Marriage and a Culturally Constructed Male Sexuality

Aamir and I were sitting outside of Sohail's grocery store when I asked him about whether he intended to get married. He seemed perplexed by my question.

"What do you mean, if I'll get married. Of course I'll get married! I want to get married...Don't I want to have children?"

"What about Sohail?" I ask.

"Sohail will get married also," Aamir replies, taking a long drag of his unfiltered cigarette.

"Will you still be with Sohail after you get married?" I ask, wanting to press the issue of how same-sex sexual relations could coexist with a desire for a marital life with a woman.

"Sohail is my jaan (life)....I could never be without him....You know, I once went to see a Sufi, a saint, whom my family visits for counsel. I did not even mention Sohail by name to Sufi sahib but just told him that I was in love with someone. Sufi sahib already knew. It was almost as if he could see in-

side my heart. He told me, 'I know you are in love with a man.' If I could, I would marry Sohail."

Sohail had joined us outside and had caught the last part of our conversation.

"How could you marry me? How would we have children?" he asked in all seriousness.

Aamir and I are silent for a minute, a little taken aback by the seriousness with which Sohail had posed the question. Aamir tries to respond equally seriously but fails.

Faisal Khan was also among the several men I became close friends with during the course of my research. Faisal had completed high school in Rawalpindi, and after several months looking for a job in the private and public sectors, took out a loan to purchase and drive a taxicab through the Pakistan prime minister's "Yellow Cab Scheme." When I met Faisal in 1994, he had been driving his taxicab for over two years and often worried about his financial situation, and with good reason. Faisal had been romantically involved with a young woman with whom he had attended high school. However, his love affair came to an abrupt end when his girlfriend's parents discovered their relationship and decided that Faisal could not provide the kind of upwardly mobile lifestyle they had hoped for their daughter. The relationship could not withstand the pressure from the parents and ended soon afterward.

It was almost a year after the relationship ended that Faisal met Salim, a junior-level executive at a local hotel in Rawalpindi. Faisal's taxicab route brought him regularly to the hotel. Over a period of several months, Faisal and Salim became friends, often spending the evenings together going for long drives in Faisal's car. However, their relationship changed on a weekend trip to a hill resort. They shared a hotel room on the trip. According to Faisal, one thing led to another, and they ended up having sex with each other.

Faisal had never had a sexual relationship with a man before Salim. When I asked Faisal about his relationship with Salim, he expressed no anxiety about being involved with another man. Instead, it was my persistent questioning of his involvement with a man that stimulated discussion on the subject.

"No, never...Never been with a man, and neither had Salim," Faisal told me as we sat in his bedroom one late evening. "I am being completely honest with you. I never thought about having sex with another man. My girlfriend

was my first love. I thought I would marry her, but her parents opposed our marriage. After my relationship ended, I just did not think I would ever be able to love someone as passionately again. ...I have only loved two people like this—my girlfriend and Salim."

"Do you think you'll get married?" I asked him as we shared a cigarette.

"I know that in America men live together as couples, but we can't do that here. Can you imagine if I was living together with Salim? If I weren't living in Pakistan, I would marry Salim. I would perform all duties of a husband and Salim, my wife."

"Would you continue your relationship with Salim after you marry?" I ask.

"Of course, my love and feelings for Salim don't have anything to do with marriage."

Sohail Agha, a consultant for the marketing of Sathi condom, points out: "In the public sphere, marital sex is the only legitimate sexual activity" (Agha, 1999: 2). In Pakistan, marriage is seen as a sacred duty and social stigma is attached to those who choose to remain single beyond a certain age. In Pakistan's conservative cultural and religious environment, even men who may eroticize a person of their own gender and *prefer* a same-sex sexual relationship would be pressured into marriage (B. Khan, 1992). Yet for all the pressures on marriage and heterosexual procreation, such societal and familial expectations do not preclude sexual relationships between men. Discussing bisexuality in India, Ramakrishnan (1991) argues that "it doesn't matter, once these [familial] duties are fulfilled, who or what you [have sex with]. So long as it is done discreetly and you don't talk about it" (4).[5]

It would be erroneous, however, to construe such expressions of same-sex sexual desire between men as a compromised expression of a homosexual desire that cannot be expressed publicly and mobilized into a sexual identity due to the cultural and religious constraints and social and religious taboos of Pakistani society. For men like Aamir, Sohail, Faisal, Salim, and Ali, having a wife and children form the basis of their status and respect within their family, kin, and community. It is not their sexual relationships and intimate friendships with men, no matter how much pleasure they may derive from them, that give meaning and validation to their *public* social life. As a writer of Pakistani male sexuality states, "the meaning and purpose of life has its root in loyalty to family, in protecting its honor and stature, in procreation, and in caring for children" (B. Khan, 1992: 94). The same author notes:

> Whether husband and wife get along with each other is strictly secondary to whether they breed well. If a husband takes care of his family's security needs and bears many children, what he does for personal sexual satisfaction is uninteresting to everyone involved, so long as he is discreet. It is certainly not discussed. It simply does not matter. It is quite irrelevant and—so long as it is kept a private matter— tolerated. (95)

In such an environment of filial and community obligations, and societal expectations, B. Khan (1992) argues that homosexual behavior is almost uninteresting:

> It does not create children, nor does it add to the potential of children in the family's resource base....Sex in general is interesting primarily because of its impact on family, rather than its potential for individual pleasure or carnal fulfillment (95).

❧

Another Genealogy of Sathi Condom:
International Development Agencies and Social Marketing Programs

A genealogy of Sathi condoms is found as much within the offices of international agencies and supranational institutions—such as the World Bank and the United Nations, which play important roles in socioeconomic development in Pakistan—as it is in the Pakistan state project of family planning. As argued in preceding sections, within the "mission" of Pakistan state agencies like the Ministry of Population Welfare, condoms and other contraceptives enter public policy through government programs and projects on family planning. What is interesting is that international development agencies, private sector agencies, and international technical consultants, who collaborated with the Pakistan state in the production of Sathi condom, leave intact the Pakistan state's constructions of the nation, family, and citizenship as essentially heterosexual.

Sathi condom was introduced in January 1987 through a project of the government of Pakistan and the United States Agency for International Development (USAID). However, the conception, marketing, and distribution of Sathi involved a complex array of institutional stakeholders that included the Ministry of Population Welfare; the National Development Finance Corporation, a semigovernment organization; Woodward Company, a private-sector corporation in Pakistan; and private-sector retail and wholesale outlets throughout urban Pakistan. Population Services International (PSI), an international marketing firm based in Washington, D.C., provided technical support for the marketing and distribution of Sathi condoms. At different stages of conception, marketing, and distribution of Sathi condoms, financial support was provided by supranational development agencies such as the World Bank, the Asian Development Bank, and the United Nations Population Fund, in addition to bilateral financial institutions, notably the Department for International Development (UK) and the German Development Bank (KfW).

The Ministry of Population Welfare was delegated by the government of Pakistan with the responsibility to manage the social marketing of Sathi condom. According to Population Services International, the primary objective of the Sathi condom project was to increase "contraceptive use by promoting family planning and expanding availability of contraceptives through the private sector" (Davies & Agha, 1997: 2). The private sector offered the advantage of a preexisting distribution network for consumer goods in urban Pakistan. The existence of local packaging, advertising, and market research firms was perceived to coalesce in enabling an effective distribution of the Sathi condom.

The Ministry of Population Welfare contracted a local marketing company, Woodward Company, to design and implement the marketing strategy of the Sathi condom. USAID procured and donated condoms that the Woodward Company packaged and sold to regional distributors for resale to wholesalers and retailers. The company was reimbursed all costs, including salaries, and received a commission on the number of condoms sold each year. The Ministry of Population Welfare also contracted with the National Development Finance Corporation to monitor Woodward's activities in the field and to oversee its financial operations, contracting procedures, and claims for reimbursement (Davies & Agha 1997). USAID contracted Population Services International to provide technical assistance, including a plan to orient all stakeholders to the social marketing plan for the Sathi condom.

Such a complexly designed social marketing program illustrates the transnational circulation of practicable models for the effective delivery of family planning goods and services through the private sector in the late twentieth century. Social marketing programs had been used for sterilization and contraceptives in Latin America (Sherris, Ravenholt, & Blackburn, 1990), and in India for the marketing of the Indian state-sponsored Nirodh condom (Ministry of Health and Family Welfare, Government of India, 1984). In Pakistan, the range of stakeholders utilized a social marketing approach to market the Sathi condom because it allowed strategic alliances and relationships between the public- and the private-sector agencies.

The specific interests of different agencies involved in the social marketing of Sathi condom varied. The Ministry of Population Welfare intended the Sathi condom to emerge as the primary method for reducing population growth through family planning and spacing of births among married couples. Woodward Company's objective was primarily market driven, and focused on increasing sales of Sathi condoms, since Woodward received a commission on each condom sold. International consultants, such as Population Services International (PSI), as discussed in the PSI reports on the marketing of the Sathi condom, were interested in the condom's financial sustainability, and related issues of the sustainability of institutional arrangements and management over time (Agha, 1998; Davies & Agha, 1997). International agencies provided logistical and substantial financial support for the Sathi condom because the management of population growth through increased contraceptive use in Pakistan was seen as facilitating sustainable development.

In spite of their varied interests, all primary actors involved in the production and marketing of the Sathi condom persisted in locating it within the Pakistan state's project of family planning without disrupting the heteronormativity implicit in such a project.

Marketing Sathi Condoms, De-Eroticizing Sex
According to Davies and Agha (1997), who served as Population Services International's consultants for the Sathi condom, most contraceptive social marketing (CSM) programs require a bridge between the government and a donor on the one hand, and commercial organizations on the other hand, in order to have a successful public-private partnership.[6] Further, Davies and Agha (1997) argue:

> The benefit of using social marketing specialists to manage CSM activities is that they understand both the public sector world of governments and donors, on the one hand, and the private sector world of commerce, on the other. In Pakistan, the SMP/PSI specialists bridge the gap between the public sector and the commercial sector, and thus help foster smooth and amicable relationships between the two sectors while managing day-to-day operations. (19)

The marketing plan for Sathi condoms, designed through a collaboration of varied national and international interests, described the target population as "men married to women of fertile age who were not protected by a modern contraceptive method" (Davies & Agha, 1997: 3). Pretesting of the condom showed a preference for orange packing and the brand name of Sathi. According to John Davies, a consultant for the project, Sathi was selected as the brand name because it suggested intimacy without an overt sexual connotation (Davies, 2002).

Promotion activities stressed the birth spacing benefits of Sathi, locating it within the exclusive domain of heterosexual marital sex and procreation. The theme used in promotion activities was "until you want another baby, rely on Sathi" (Davies & Agha, 1997: 4). However, print and visual media were not fully utilized to market and advertise the condom because of fears of protests from religious and conservative groups opposed to an open discussion of sexuality and contraceptive use. The Ministry of Population Welfare buckled under such perceived pressure and potential backlash and rejected plans to advertise the Sathi condom on state-controlled television and radio (Davies & Agha, 1997).

As a result, Woodward Company focused promotions efforts at the retail level, and used forty USAID-funded salesmen to introduce Sathi to retailers in each community by offering prizes for the best displays of Sathi condoms in retail outlets. Importantly, "these retail promotions treated Sathi just like other consumer products, not as a product that is unusual or sensitive" (Davies & Agha, 1997: 3-4). Woodward Company distributed the condom through the same networks that it had utilized for its other consumer products. These regional distributors, located in 110 cities in Pakistan, sold the condoms to wholesalers and retailers in their region.

Within just one year, over 30 million Sathi condoms had been sold. The number increased to 34 million in 1988 and to 44 million in 1989 (Davies & Agha, 1997). The usage increased dramatically to 74 million in 1990, and decreased only slightly to 73 million in 1991. The 1990-91 Demographic and Health Survey of the Government of Pakistan attributes the success of the Sathi condom to active social marketing. Davies and Agha offer an alternative explanation for the success of Sathi, especially during the initial years of its introduction in the Pakistani market. According to Davies and Agha (1997):

> Contrary to fears often expressed in Pakistan, overt display of condoms in thousands of stores in rich and poor areas, and some advertising in newspapers, resulted in very little backlash. By packaging and promoting *Sathi just like other commercial products, such as soap or cigarettes, Sathi* was quickly accepted as one of those products. (16) [Emphasis added]

Sathi condom's enormous initial success then, can be attributed in large part to its marketing as any other commercial product. Sathi condom was de-eroticized to signify a generalized commercial product, rather than a specific product of erotic desire and pleasure.

William Mazzarella's excellent essay on the marketing of the KamaSutra condoms in Bombay in India (Mazzarella, 2001) illuminates additional cultural and national contexts of condom usage in the South Asian region. According to Mazzarella, the KamaSutra condom "was launched at a time when the Indian government had adapted the IMF imposed regime of economic liberalization, and increased consumerism in the Indian middle class" (168). KamaSutra condoms offered "an aestheticized version of national development and the public sphere that focused on consumer goods as the markers of individual self-realization and collective progress" (168). The advertising for KamaSutra condom was intended to develop

> images that would elicit an aesthetic response to the new "liberalizing" dispensation, thus legitimizing it on a level more libidinally powerful than the abstractions of economic discourse. (168-9)

Unlike the marketing of Sathi condom in Pakistan, KamaSutra condom was positioned as a luxury product, and "its eroticized packaging spoke to the aspirations of the consumerist *avant garde*" (Mazzarella, 2001: 169).

The marketing for KamaSutra condom in India could not be more different from the cultural and religious environment in which the Sathi condom was marketed in Pakistan. Promotions in the print media constituted a significant component for the advertisement for the KamaSutra condom in India. Mazzaralla's wonderful description of an advertisement for KamaSutra condoms bears repeating at length. The print ads consisted of

> blue tinted photographs of a half-clad couple, clutching each other in a variety of urgently passionate poses. The aesthetic parameters were clearly derived from the visual repertoire of fashion shoots and the glossier end of rock videos, suggesting candidly captured yet carefully stylized moments. The man was invariably positioned in a supporting role as the ardent source of the female model's pleasure. Both of them had closed eyes, the man's face usually half-hidden, while the woman's head was thrown back, suggesting submission to a pleasure heightened by the discerning deployment of a *KamaSutra* condom. Each ad featured one of a series of quotations from the text of the *KamaSutra* itself, by ways of hints for the sophisticated lover. In at least one case, the text directly implied that the acquisition of the product might be the key to a woman's desire....The man should do whatever the girl takes most delight in, and he should get for her, whatever she may have a desire to possess. (172-3)

According to Mazzaralla, this conceptualization of premium condoms in India dissociated condoms from both the state project of family planning and discourses on HIV/AIDS. According to one account of the design and marketing of KamaSutra, the intention was to distance KamaSutra from prior family planning initiatives, "widely resisted by the urban middle class, especially given the violent experience of authoritarian actions by Indira Gandhi during the emergency of 1975–1977" (Mazzarella, 2001, 180) when forced sterilization took place on a mass scale. Equally, KamaSutra was dissociated from AIDS because of the perceived implication that one's lifestyle somehow connoted a vulnerability of contracting the AIDS virus.

The marketing of KamaSutra stands in stark contrast to the advertisements for Sathi condoms in Pakistan. Family planning initiatives in Pakistan focus on a silhouette of a woman with her head covered, a man, and two children—a boy and a girl, with the caption *hum do hamare do* (two people, two children). Government-dispensed contraceptives, including condoms, were intended by the state to regulate sexual activity within the exclusive context of a religiously ordained, heterosexual union between a man and a woman. The varied institutional interests and stakeholders involved in the marketing of the Sathi condom built on the Pakistan state's project and marketed Sathi condom primarily to low-income married couples.

Where private sector advertising agencies in India successfully and creatively conceived an erotically charged print ad campaign for the KamaSutra condom, social marketing for the Sathi condom in Pakistan attempted to de-eroticize the condom, locating it as a generalized consumer product. Yet there is something subversive about naming the condom *Sathi*. Pakistani men often refer to close male friends as their Sathi. Just as KamaSutra invoked a recognizable, indigenous, and ancient "Indian treatise on the science of the senses" (Mazzarella, 2001, 174), Sathi too invoked images of a culturally constructed male sexuality, in which *sathi* (friend) is not just platonic, but the object of one's erotic desire and pleasure.

In the following section, I continue the analysis of same-sex sexual desire among men, through the lens of intimate male friendships. I argue that for a segment of Pakistani men, sexual male friendships, sometimes defined as *sathi*, participated in bringing Sathi condom out from the exclusive domain of family planning and heterosexual and procreative marital sex, into an inclusive domain of erotic desire within intimate male friendships.

Re-Eroticizing Sathi Condom: Intimate Friendships among Men

There are several words in Urdu used interchangeably for "friend," among them *dost, humsafar, Sathi,* and *yaar*. The narrative below of a South Asian man most poignantly situates intimate male friendships within the realm of erotic desire.

> Over the past few years I have come to realize that my meandering path through romance, sexual liaisons, and friendship has been, and still is, but a search for a singular relationship that can encompass all three of these elements. Such a bond is embodied in the concept of *yaari*. A *yaar* is an individual with whom one feels a deep, almost intangible connection....For me a *yaar* embodies elements of both a friend and a lover, and I yearn for just such a connection with a man in my life....There is really no English equivalent for this concept, no word that approaches its breadth and depth. *Friend* is not enough. *Buddy* is superficial, reeks of Budweiser beers and backslapping in bars....A world of romantic images revolves around *yaari*. There are tales of *yaars* dying for one another. Even a wife must many a time take a backseat to a man's *yaar*. (Ayyar, 1993: 167)

Narratives of friendships, such as the one below, similarly blur the line between platonic friendships and intimate, eroticized friendships between men:

> We were friends for a long time and then started flirting and making jokes about how attractive we found each other....One evening we were at his house and were lying on his bed and talking. The next thing I knew we were hugging madly. We took each other's clothes off and touched for hours. Our affair continued for a year....Emotionally we were close as any lovers (ABVA, 1991, p. 8).

Joel Hencken (1984) underscores the permissibility of such relationships in his essay on homosexual behaviors that preclude homosexual labeling. According to Hencken:

> For more involved relationships, "special friendships" and love may be emphasized so that the relationship is seen as an expression of unique feelings for the partner that have no implications for sexual identity. (56)

Lawrence Cohen, writing about the exchange of Holi (Hindu festival of color) greeting cards among Hindu men in the city of Banaras in India, states that the men he interviewed spoke "not only of play...but of *pyar mohabbat*, of love and of the passions of the heart" (Cohen, 1995: 418). Cohen notes that drawings of an erect phallus did not refer to the world of the "the doer and the done to." Instead, "he [the sender] had drawn it from life and was offering it, as Penis, to another. *Holi* was here the possibility of penetration being a gift" (Cohen, 1995: 418). B. Khan (1992) expresses a similar romanticized account of relationships between men in South Asia when he states:

> Love between men is, in fact, exalted, and tenderness, affection, and deep friendships are not uncommon. Unlike the macho backslap that passes for camaraderie in the West, men frequently hold hands while walking, and it is not uncommon to see men embracing. (B. Khan, 1992: 99)

Intimate male friendships become defined in such eroticized ways, in part, because of the cultural permissibility of intense male bonding that is expressed in single-sex institutions such as schools, or through socialization that brings together young men and creates gendered public cultures of leisure activities, entertainment, sociality, and living; that is, eating, working, and sleeping together. The permissibility of same-sex sexual desire in intimate friendships may be due to "the close emotional bonding and physical affection between male friends while discouraging premarital heterosexual social life, and the prevalence of boarding schools and late arranged marriage ages" (Dynes & Donaldson, 1992: xii). Homosociality is also culturally reinforced, exalted, and glorified in South Asian popular culture, notably Hindu films, the primary source of entertainment for middle- and low-income families in general and men in particular in India and Pakistan. The theme of several popular films centers on the almost sacredness of male friendships, in which men willingly sacrifice the love of their beloved (a woman) for the love of their friend (a man). An anthropologist who lived with a Tamil family in southern India during the 1980s suggests that such themes in Indian mainstream feature films were continually reproduced in the social relations and vice versa (Trawick, 1992). This homosociality also extends to poetry and popular songs that "talk of undying friendship between men [and] are part of the repertoire of popular verse" (B. Khan, 1992: 99). According to an eighteenth-century Urdu poet, Abru, "He who avoids the boy and desires the woman is not in love but a man of lust" (Naim, 1979: 130).

The cultural acceptance and social reinforcement of homosociality and male bonding contributes to the lack of gender anxiety about sex between close male friends. Cohen states that the intense homosociality is defined not through "homosexual panic but through mutuality and *dosti* (friendship)" (Cohen, 1995: 417). It may be, as Cohen suggests, that homosociality holds the potential to collapse playfulness and penetration into a single desire. However, in this context, sexual activity is transformed into a *khel* or *masti*, which allows sex to be situated within the domain of a friendship with flexible boundaries. Cohen, for instance, notes:

> Different men may articulate the boundaries of friendship and play differently....The boys and men who play around with friends their own age and of similar backgrounds must negotiate this mutual terrain of play. (1995: 417)

Despite the gendered spaces of male sociality and the permissibility of eroticized friendships and their reinforcement in popular culture, these relationships do not replace or erase the desire for a heterosexual marital relationship. Instead, intimate male friendships coexist with the ideals of marriage, family, and children. The seeming impossibility of reconciling the two is belied by the everyday negotiations of sexual desire, with larger societal and familial expectations regarding heterosexual marriage and procreation.

Conclusion: Attitudes toward Condom Usage among Punjabi Men

In spite of the availability of a local interpretive framework for re-eroticizing the Sathi condom and breaking it free from the narrow confines of a heteronormative Pakistan state ideology, attitudes toward actual condom usage vary considerably among the Punjabi men I met during the course of my research. Recall the vignette with which I begin this essay. Aamir had shown his reluctance to use condoms, even jokingly telling his sexual partner, Sohail: "What, are you worried you'll get pregnant? You know I don't like wearing Sathi. I'll use it when I get married...I don't feel anything when I wear it....*bilkul maza nahi aata* (I feel absolutely no pleasure)...but I'll wear it for you." Although Aamir's reluctance can be read as a matter of aesthetics and sexual pleasure, it is equally indicative of an association that men like Aamir make between condoms, procreation, and marital sex. With condom usage relegated to family planning, procreation, and marital sex, same-sex sexual relationships come to occupy a less vigilantly regulated space vis-à-vis condom usage.

This is not to argue that the men included in my research used condoms reluctantly, if at all, while having sex with other men. Men like Faisal did in fact associate condom usage with safe sex. When I asked Faisal whether he used condoms while having sex with Salim, he answered without a moment's hesitation: "Of course, although you know, it never really comes up. Salim always carries Sathi with him, and he puts it on before we have sex. But we never really talk about it." Such attitudes toward condom usage suggest the limits of the discourse on sexuality among a segment of Pakistani men. While male sexual partners might well perceive condom usage as being necessary, the act of using condoms is devoid of elaborate verbal mediation. It is, if you will, simply understood that condoms need to be used for safe sex.

Yet perhaps the most startling and disturbing of all attitudes toward condom usage came from Reza, when we met for dinner one evening. Reza had recently started working as a receptionist at a local hotel, but planned to return to school for his undergraduate degree in a couple of years. Reza lived with his maternal grandparents, father and mother, and a younger sister in the heart of Rawalpindi city. Lacking the private space in which to entertain his partner, Javed, they often met at an inexpensive motel, or at Javed's home when Javed's family was away.

We had been chatting about his relationship with Javed, when I asked him whether he used condoms. Reza suddenly became uncomfortable, fidgeting in his chair and barely making any eye contact with me. Reza had hesitated before saying. "I want to, really I do; but Javed just doesn't listen. I mean, I told him that I wouldn't have sex without Sathi, but he just kept refusing to use one. The other day, I refused to have sex if he didn't wear Sathi. I could see Javed was becoming more and more agitated and angry....I was really scared of what he might do if I refused... so I let him."

Javed's violent refusal is difficult to understand and analyze. I had minimal interaction with Javed and never quite reached the level of friendship with him to engage in a candid discussion of his attitude toward condom usage. Still, I see Javed's refusal as an important testament to the inaccessibility of global discourses on safe sex and HIV/AIDS prevention within certain groups that persist in practicing high-risk sexual activities. Simply because Sathi finds a place in the interpretive framework of eroticized male friendships and sexual relationships does not necessarily translate into its usage within such sexual relationships. The barrier to safer sex practices might well be explained through the aesthetic of using condoms, and their perceived effect on constraining the active partner's sexual pleasure. Equally, though, Javed's reaction speaks to the inequality and differential power relations that can characterize sexual relationships between men.

There is enormous variability in the formation of a sexual self, family structure, and marital relations across socioeconomic class, ethnicity, region, and religious locations in Pakistan. As such, any analysis of the constructions of intimate male relationships and same-sex sexual desire need to be situated and contextualized within the specificity of myriad social positions and locations. In this essay, I have attempted to show the intersection of a specific group of lower-middle-class single men from the ethnolinguistic Punjabi community in urban Pakistan, with state ideologies and practices of family planning during the 1990s. All of these men were in involved in intimate and erotic sexual friendships with other men. Yet they situated themselves within the state project of family planning and contraceptive usage rather than locate themselves outside of it.

In their construction of sexuality, men like Aamir, Sohail, Salim, Faisal, Reza, and Ali were able to form and sustain intimate sexual relationships with other men, while simultaneously adhering to societal and familial expectations and their own desire for marriage. This everyday renegotiation of same-sex sexual desire with societal and familial expectations becomes visible in their creative appropriation of the heteronormative conception and marketing of the Sathi condom. It allows them to enter the story of the Sathi condom, and indeed, for the Sathi condom to enter their lives, through the prism of same-sex sexual desire rather than marital and procreative sex. The preceding ethnographic analysis has significant implications for ethnographic studies and public policy interventions in areas of sexual health, family planning, and population control in cultural and national contexts where western paradigms of sexuality are only one of myriad interpretative frameworks for understanding erotic desire and male sexuality.

Acknowledgments

The essay has benefited from the intellectual support and generous advice from Linda-Anne Rebhun, Matthew Nelson, William Mazzaralla, Eric Worby, and Kamari Clarke. Safiya Aftab, a close friend and a valued interlocutor in my research, provided valuable research support in Pakistan. I would also like to acknowledge BAIA (Basic AIDS Information and Awareness Group) in Islamabad, and the Sustainable Development Policy Institute (SDPI) in Islamabad in providing logistical and institutional support during the period of my field research on HIV/AIDS and male sexual health from 1993 to 1997. I am thankful and grateful to the editors of this volume, especially Jessamyn Neuhaus, for their persistence, support, and patience as I worked on this essay. Finally, I am grateful for the opportunity this research provided me to meet and learn from the life experiences of the men included in this essay. I remain indebted to them for their friendship and infallible trust in me as I sometimes intrusively delved into their personal lives.

Notes

[1] All names used throughout the essay are pseudonyms. In keeping with established protocol for confidentiality in social science research, I have changed the names and certain identifying details of all interlocutors discussed in this essay.

[2] Throughout the essay, the discussion and analysis of male sexuality in Pakistan, a predominantly Muslim country, focuses on cultural and not explicitly *religious* frameworks. The decision to exclude a separate discussion of religion in the everyday life of men included in this essay is a deliberate strategy for two main reasons: First, although all interlocutors are practicing Muslims—belonging to the dominant Sunni sect of Islam—religion never came up as a distinct subject of discussion in my conversations and interviews. For these men, religion is an irreducible and nonnegotiable facet of identity and community life. Indeed, religion is present in all facets of social life. In the realm of same-sex relationships, religion is in the background but not forgotten. For example, most men included in this research abstained from sexual intercourse during the month of Ramadan, when Muslims fast from sunrise to sunset. These men also avoided sexual relations during the call to prayers five times a day. Such religious prohibitions against all sexual relations were implicitly understood but seldom articulated verbally.

Second, most ethnographic analyses of Pakistanis and the Pakistani Diaspora privilege religion as the primary—and often as the only—site for constructing identity, community, and nationhood. In this essay, I was especially keen to find new ways to write about Pakistanis in the contemporary moment that were not dependent on discourses of secularism and religion. That said, it will be important for future research on male sexual health and same-sex desire—particularly in Pakistan and in other Muslim countries, and among Muslim groups—to explore the intersection of religion with constructions of male sexuality. Future studies might consider the religious prohibitions and sanctions against public admission and expression of same-sex desire. Such research is critical. In Pakistan, as is the case in most Muslim countries, public admission of homosexuality is a punishable crime, and subject to severe legal, social, and familial sanctions.

For important discussions of homosexuality/same-sex desire and Islam, please see Jamal, A. (2001), "The Story of Lot and the Quran's Perception of the Morality of Same-Sex Sexuality" in the *Journal of Homosexuality,* 4(1): 1; and Nahas, O. (2001). *Islam en Homoseksualiteit.* Amsterdam: Bulaaq.

[3] In recent years, the culture of "down-low" suggests a similar culturally conceived male sexuality among African-American men in the United States. The down-low refers to same-sex relationships between heterosexual, married African-American men. Notably, these men engage in sex with other men without self-identification as homosexual or even bisexual. The down-low culture of male sociality is being linked to the increased incidence of HIV infections among heterosexual African-American women who are married to men on the down low. For an autobiographical account of the down-low culture, please see King, J. L. (2004). *On the Down Low: A Journey into the Lives of "Straight" Black Men Who Sleep with Men.*

New York, Broadway Publishers. For a sociological discussion of same-sex sexual behavior among American men who do not self-identity as homosexual or bisexual, please see Humphreys, L. (1970). *Tearoom Trade: Impersonal Sex in Public Places*. Chicago: Aldine Press.

[4] For important theoretical discussions of cultural constructions of male sexuality, please see the follow essays: Hencken, J. D. (1984). "Conceptualizations of Homosexual Behavior Which Preclude Homosexual Self-labeling." *Journal of Homosexuality*, 9(4), 53–63; Blumstein, P., & Schwartz, P. (1990). Intimate Relationships and the Creation of Sexuality. In D. P. McWhirter (Ed.), *Homosexuality/Heterosexuality: Concepts of Sexual Orientation*.New York: Oxford; Byne, W. (1997). "Why We Cannot Conclude that Sexual Orientation Is Primarily a Biological Phenomena." *Journal of Homosexuality*, 34(1), 73–80; De Cecco, J. P., & Elia, J. P. (1993). "A Critique and Synthesis of Biological Essentialism and Social Constructionist Views of Sexuality and Gender." *Journal of Homosexuality*, 24(3/4), 1–26.

[5] In several places in this essay, I draw on analyses and discussions of male sexuality in India to inform the discussion of male same-sex desire in Pakistan. The slippage between India and Pakistan is intentional. The inclusion of India-centered research on male sexuality in an essay about Pakistani men is intended to position sexuality as an important site for the cultural convergence between postcolonial India and Pakistan. Equally, given the paucity of research on male sexuality in contemporary Pakistan, it was important to refer to studies of male same-sex desire in India because of the persistence of shared cultural idioms of desire and sexuality that transcend the geographical borders of the postcolonial South Asian nation-states.

[6] Population Services International (PSI) separates the marketing of the Sathi condom in Pakistan into three distinct stages: one, implementation by a commercial marketing firm (1987–1990); two, the development of a management committee, including representatives of government, international donors, Pakistani private sector firms, and social marketers (1991–1993); and three, management by social marketing specialists (1994–1996). In all three stages: A partnership between a local social marketing firm and an international social marketing firm [was perceived by PSI] to be an appropriate way of organizing and managing a large-scale program which trains private doctors and pharmacists about the use of IUDs and injectable contraceptives. (Davies & Agha, 1997: 19)

Bibliography

Abdul, H. A., Cleland, J., & Mansoor, U. H. B. (1997). Preliminary report. *Pakistan Fertility and Family Planning Survey, 1996–97*.

Afzal, A. (1995). Public policy limitations: The individual, the family, and AIDS in Pakistan. *Development*, 2: 61–63.

Agha, S. (1998). Contraceptive social marketing in Pakistan: Assessing the impact of the 1991 condom price increases on sales and consumption. *Working Paper No. 14*. Washington, D.C.: PSI Research Division.

———. (1999). Sexual behavior of truck drivers in Pakistan: Implications for AIDS prevention programs. *Working Paper No. 24*. Washington, D.C.: PSI Research Division.

AIDS Bhedbhav Virodhi Andolan (ABVA). (1991). *Less than gay: A citizens' report on the status of homosexuality in India*. New Delhi: Author.

Alexander, M. J. (1997). Erotic autonomy as a politics of decolonization: an anatomy of feminist and state practice in the Bahamas tourist economy. In M. J. Alexander & C. T. Mohanty (Eds.), *Feminist genealogies, colonial legacies, democratic futures* (p. 84). New York: Routledge.

Ayyar, R. (1993). Yaari. In Rakesh Ratti (Ed.), *A lotus of another color: An unfolding of the south Asian gay and lesbian experience*. Boston: Alyson Publications.

Blumstein, P., & Schwartz, P. (1990). Intimate relationships and the creation of sexuality. In David P. McWhirter (Ed.), *Homosexuality/Heterosexuality: Concepts of sexual orientation*. New York: Oxford University Press.

Byne, W. (1997). Why we cannot conclude that sexual orientation is primarily a biological phenomena. *Journal of Homosexuality, 34*(1): 73–80.

Carrier, J. M. (1976). Cultural factors affecting urban Mexican male homosexual behavior. *Archives of Sexual Behavior, 5*(2): 103–124.

Cernada, G. P., & Bob, U. (1992). Pakistan's fertility and family planning: Future directions. *Journal of Family Welfare, 38*(3): 49–56.

Cohen, L. (1995). *Holi* in Banaras and the Mahaland of modernity. *Gay and Lesbian Quarterly (GLQ), 2*: 399–424.

Davies, J. (2002). Personal communication, October 21.

Davies, J., & Agha, S. (1997). Ten years of contraceptive social marketing in Pakistan: An assessment of management, outputs, effects, costs and cost-efficiency, 1987–1996. *Working Paper No. 7.* Washington, D.C.: PSI Research Division.

Davies, J., & Louis, T. D. J. (1977). Assessing the impact of a social marketing program: Preethi in Sri Lanka. *Studies in Family Planning, 8*(4): 82–90.

De Cecco, J. P., & Elia, J. P. (1991). A critique and synthesis of biological essentialism and social constructionist views of sexuality and gender. *Journal of Homosexuality, 24*(3/4), 1–26.

Dynes W. & Donaldson S., (Eds.) (1992). *Asian homosexuality.* New York: Taylor & Francis.

Dynes, W. & Donaldson, S., (Eds.) (1992). *History of homosexuality in Europe and America.* New York and London: Garland Publishing.

Gopinath, G. (1997). Nostalgia, desire, disapora: South Asian sexualities in motion. *Positions,* 5(2): 467–489.

Hencken, J. D. (1984). Conceptualizations of homosexual behavior which preclude homosexual self-labeling. *Journal of Homosexuality,* 9(4): 53–63.

Humphreys, L. (1970). *Tearoom trade: Impersonal sex in public places.* Chicago: Aldine Press.

Jamal, A. (2001). The story of Lot and the Qur'an's perception of the morality of same-sex sexuality. *Journal of Homosexuality,* 4(1): 1–88.

Khan, B. (1992). Not-so-gay life in Karachi: A view of a Pakistani living in Toronto. In A. Schmitt & J. Sofer (Eds.), *Sexuality and eroticism among males in Moslem societies.* New York: Haworth Press.

Khan, S. (1997a). Observations on male to male sexual behaviors in India and Bangladesh. In Naz Foundation, *Perspectives on males who have sex with males in India and Bangladesh*. London: Naz Foundation.

———. (1997b). Under the blanket: Bisexualities and AIDS in India. In Naz Foundation, *Perspectives on males who have sex with males in India and Bangladesh*. London: Naz Foundation.

———. (1997c). Cultural constructions of male sexualities in India. In Naz Foundation, *Perspectives on males who have sex with males in India and Bangladesh*. London: Naz Foundation.

Lancaster, R. N. (1988). Subject honor and object shame: the construction of male homosexuality and stigma in Nicaragua. *Ethnology*, 27(2): 111–125.

Maudlin, W. P., & Ross, J. A. (1994). Prospects and programs for fertility reduction, 1990–2015. *Studies in Family Planning*, 25(2): 77–95.

Mazzarella, W. (2001). Citizens have sex, consumers make love: Marketing KamaSutra condoms in Bombay. In B. Moeran (Ed.), *Asian media productions*. Surrey, UK: Curzon Press.

Ministry of Health and Family Welfare. (1984). *Nirodh program: A pioneering social marketing project in India*. New Delhi: November.

Ministry of Population Welfare. (2002). Ministry of Population Welfare web site: *www.mopw.gov.pk*. Islamabad: Government of Pakistan.

Nahas, O. (2001). *Islam en Homoseksualiteit*. Amsterdam: Bulaaq.

Naim, C. M. (1979). The theme of homosexual love in pre-modern Urdu poetry. In Mohammad Umar Memon (Ed.), *Studies in the Urdu Ghazal and prose fiction*. University of Wisconsin Publication Series, Publication No. 5. Madison: University of Wisconsin Press.

Parker, R. (1986). Masculinity, femininity, and homosexuality: On the anthropological interpretation of sexual meanings in Brazil. In E. Blackwood (Ed.), *The many faces of homosexuality: Anthropological approaches to homosexual behavior* (pp. 155–163). New York: Harrington Park Press.

———. (1999). *Beneath the equator: Cultures of desire, male homosexuality, and emerging gay communities in Brazil.* New York: Routledge.

Population Welfare Division. (1986). *Pakistan contraceptive prevalence survey.* Islamabad: Planning Department, Government of Pakistan.

Ramakrishnan. (1991). Bisexuality: Identities, behaviors and politics. *Trikone,* April.

Rosen, J., & Conly, S. (1996). The Pakistan population program: The challenge ahead. *Country Studies Series #3.* Washington, D.C.: Population Action International.

Sathar, Z. A. (1993). The much awaited fertility decline in Pakistan: Wishful thinking or reality? *International Family Planning Perspectives, 19*(4): 142–146.

Sherris, J., Ravenholt, B. and Blackburn, R. (1990). Contraceptive social marketing: Lessons from experience. *Population Reports, Series J, No. 30*: 773–812.

Stein, T. S. (1997). Deconstructing sexual orientation: Understanding the phenomena of sexual orientation. *Journal of Homosexuality, 34*(1): 81–86.

Sultan, M., Cleland, J. G., & Ali, M. M. (2002). Assessment of a new approach to family planning services in rural Pakistan. *American Journal of Public Health, 92*(7): 11–68.

Taylor, C. L. (1986). Mexican male homosexual interaction in public contexts. In E. Blackwood (Ed.) *The many faces of homosexuality: Anthropological approaches to homosexual behavior* (pp. 117–136). New York: Harrington Park Press.

Trawick, M. (1992). *Notes on love in a Tamil family.* Berkeley: University of California Press.

Weinberg, T. S. (1978). On 'doing' and 'being' gay: Sexual behavior and homosexual male identity. *Journal of Homosexuality, 4*(9): 143–156.

• CHAPTER SIXTEEN •

The Colors of the Condom: Benetton's Seductive Images

Jill Scott

In the early 1990s when the panic over an AIDS epidemic was just peaking, Benetton's hip and trendy lifestyle magazine, *COLORS*, ran an article on the "colors of the condom," including a centerfold featuring larger-than-life pictures of an array of brilliant condoms such as "The Banana," "The Spiked," "Black Licorice," "Teddy," "Gargoyle," and even condoms for flower arrangers. With their fun names, cool colors, and polyvocality, these images included all the traits of Benetton's target market of global youth, promising the nostalgia of carefree sex but also political correctness through the promotion of safe sex. This mixed message speaks to the paradoxes of postmodern society—an addiction to authenticity, the appropriation of Otherness through Benetton's colorful and exoticized bodies, and ultimately the failure to see the connection between "color" and race.

This chapter will explore the problematic role of the condom as a veil that protects and hides, promises the fulfillment of desire and promotes seduction, and yet denies the referent itself, the body—healthy or diseased, rich or poor, black or white. Through a theoretical framework based on Baudrillard's concept of *seduction*, it will be argued that the condom constructed through the media discourse of the 1990s is self-referential, self-reflexive, and ultimately self-seductive. The Phallus, the Lacanian symbol of "Truth," disappears behind the veil of the condom and the penis itself becomes an empty signifier, emasculated and without reference.[1] The condom is thus a postmodern smokescreen that masks the "real" and fashions personality as a meaningless pastiche.[2] The second focus of the chapter rests on the bitter irony of Benetton's condoms: The attempt to appropriate and exoticize Otherness through color and difference veils the harsh reality that the vast majority of the people dying from AIDS, a disease barely mentioned by Benetton, are people of color.

Benetton and the Culture of Consumption

Before coming to the analysis of its portrayal of condoms, let us first examine Benetton's representational practices. The company's ad campaign caused enormous controversy in the early 1990s, but it did not actually initiate anything new. In fact, the ads participated in a trend in advertising that began with the dawn of modernity—that of distancing the sign from the referent. The product is no longer front and center in the frame but plays a peripheral role in a semiotic collage assembled to create a mood or invoke a feeling. The sun setting behind a distant mountain becomes a romantic backdrop for a car or a cigarette, and the consumer is invited to invest in the sexiness of the scene. Common scenarios involve pristine nature, exotic peoples, and locales that afford the viewer a sense of colonial power. The most ubiquitous image of consumer manipulation, however, remains the all-American blonde babe. Sex sells.

Pictures of good-looking people, young people, the exposure of the body together with a hint of a garment—a T-shirt, handbag, jeans unbuttoned at the waist—have been the norm for some time. Though feminists have waged war on the denigration of women and staged a serious critique against their exploitation in ads, these voices have remained at the margin and have played a relatively minor role in influencing consumer habits. The public eye has become complacent and almost accepting of vague eroticism and odd suggestiveness in ads for everything from clothes and cars to perfume, jewelry, and of course, condoms. So why is it that Benetton's sensationalist ad campaigns provoked the ire of governments, institutions, activists, and the Catholic Church?

Perhaps the answer lies in Benetton's calculated risk in taking advertising to a radical new level. Its campaign erased the referent—knitwear fashions—altogether and replaced it with a series of disturbing images—of violence, terrorism, racial stereotypes, homosexuality—many of which were deemed too shocking for general audiences. It seems that distancing the referent is perceived as mildly amusing and playfully erotic, in the way that a scantily clad woman is said to be more seductive than a naked female body. The imagination may be more evocative than the image, but removing the referent entirely is suspect. Benetton's self-conscious and self-referential ads make the public much more aware of the "targeting" and manipulation that takes place in a typical ad campaign, where the product is at least vaguely present.[3]

From the outset of its new advertising strategy, launched in 1991, Benetton was frank about its mission. Ever since it introduced its 1985 slogan

"United Colors of Benetton," the company's aim had been to promote racial harmony and world peace, which it pursued through playful photos of multiracial youths dressed in Benetton attire. With the arrival of the shocking new ads, the message had changed. In response to the critique of the ads, the company maintained that its intention all along was "not to sell sweaters": "We're not that stupid," claimed spokesperson Peter Fressola. "We're doing corporate communication." He maintained that the real concern of the company was to raise awareness and compassion around a number of key social issues (Squiers, 1992, 18). Contradicting these statements, Luciano Benetton admitted that the advertising campaign had a "traditional function...to make Benetton known around the world and to introduce the product to consumers" (Sischy, 1992, 69). In its magazine, *COLORS*, the company asserted, however, that the form of communication it promoted with its sensational images would be "more useful to society" (Fall/Winter 1992, 2).[4]

Benetton claimed that it was concerned with its social responsibility to global problems such as the AIDS crisis, environmental disaster, political violence, war, exile, and natural catastrophe. As a major international corporation with the means to reach a large audience, it would use its ads in a different way. Few people were convinced by this argument—images of a tattooed arm bearing the letters "HIV," a man dying of AIDS, a duck coated with oil from an ocean spill, or the suffering of small black children were called "a serious misappropriation of human misery" (Colombo, 1993, 74). If Benetton wanted only to raise awareness of key issues such as violence and the environment, why then the strategic placement of its logo in a distinctive green box at the edge of each photo? Product placement had been replaced with name-brand recognition, and Benetton's new ads were all about logo and hype. The logo is the ultimate form of cultural capital, permeating every aspect of our society, from toilet paper to condoms, and is central to our politics of identity. "As we buy, wear, and eat logos," claims Susan Willis (1983), "we become the henchmen and admen of the corporations, defining ourselves with respect to the social standing of the various corporations" (133). Similarly, Joanne Finkelstein (1991) theorizes shopping as a means of simulating the subject, indeed as a form of shopping for the self. She claims that ads such as Benetton's drive us to seek "the iconic imitation of the successful, powerful, rich, famous, beautiful, youthful and talented" (172). Ironically, it is precisely through this endless consumption of goods that the subject itself is lost in a perpetual simulation, as Lauren Langman (1992) asserts: "If the subject is not dead, s/he is more likely decentered, fragmented, and differentially expressed and experienced depending on context"

(67). The self becomes as far removed from its referent as Benetton's clothes are from their advertising practices.

Benetton's rhetoric of social responsibility was viewed as nothing more than a cheap way to profit from human misery. The target audience of eighteen- to thirty-four-year-olds traditionally relishes rebellious behavior and the rejection of conservative social values such as those held by governments and the Catholic Church (the chief critics of the campaign). Thus, purchasing a colorful wool sweater fashioned by Benetton was no longer about use-value or exchange-value but about political-value—that is, an opportunity to participate in a revolution. This all translated into phenomenal economic success for a clothing company.

Founded in 1965 as a family business by Luciano Benetton and three of his siblings, the company expanded over two decades to become a global operation worth more than $2 billion, producing over 80 million items of clothing every year. It peaked at approximately seven thousand franchises in over one hundred countries and approached the name-brand recognition of Coca-Cola at the height of its advertising scandals (O'Leary, 1992, 28). In 1984, award-winning photographer Oliviero Toscani joined the company to head its international advertising campaign, and by 1991 his budget had risen to $80 million. It was at this point that the company shifted its emphasis from sales to pedagogy, or so it claimed.

Benetton had become the world's largest consumer of virgin wool and produced mountains of knitwear and other garments for a fashion-conscious public. Consumers hungry for a new identity built around the neoliberal slogans about the environment, racial politics, and the like were duped into the naive assumption that they could save the world by buying Benetton products. On the contrary, such purchases would only continue the harmful practices the company had itself been preaching against. Benetton's consumption of raw materials to feed First World markets for new clothes only further damaged fragile ecosystems and depleted the Earth of precious resources. Moreover, the company's millions of dollars of sponsorship in Formula One auto racing further contradicted its environmental mandate.

All the while placing ads about racial harmony, Benetton continued to exploit cheap labor markets in poor countries, where most workers are inevitably people of color. The irony of the ads featuring bodies of all different races and ethnicities is that most of these groups have historically been the victims of colonialism and continue to be economically disadvantaged such that they are in all likelihood unable to participate in the consumption practices promoted by Benetton. On top of this, the company began to encourage people to give their old clothes to charity, the irony of which is that this generous philanthropic act would only give birth to an empty closet yearning for more new fashions—Benetton's, of course. In short, the so-called social responsibility of the ad campaign did little more than line the company's own pockets. The scandals and controversy around the ads was a win/win situation for Benetton—the more sensational and shocking the pictures, the more they were debated in the media and on the street, the more their name-brand recognition grew.

The Condom Ad That Is Not a Condom Ad
Condoms figure largely in one such ad, though Benetton is not of course in the business of selling condoms. We see life-size silhouettes of multicolored condoms in different sizes and shapes suspended in midair like fish floating in water. The sheaths are shown stretched out with the distinctive tapered tip veiling an imaginary penis. Because the condoms are translucent, with only a hint of muted pastel tones, they appear to fade into the background, and the most distinctive image we are left with is the round O shape of the rubber opening. This image is suggestive of a vaginal opening or an ovum waiting to be fertilized. Seen from a distance, one might mistake the condoms for a collection of sperm and eggs. The ad is characteristic of Toscani's trademark ambiguity, most obvious in photographs such as the priest kissing a nun, a black woman with a white baby at her breast, or two hands, one black and one white, connected by handcuffs. The condom image promotes both contraception in the form of the condom and fertility in the form of the egg. It contains another twofold message—that of safe sex through the protective condom and that of free love, the kind that leads to conception.

As with all of Toscani's creations, we find a small green box with the logo "United Colors of Benetton" placed at the far right edge of the ad. This logo is more an icon than a message *per se*, because it has become so familiar to the viewing public that it is internalized as a unit rather than a syntactical sequence of words. Nevertheless, it plays an important role in the semiology of the condom collage. In this case the "United Colors" refers polysemically to the actual colors of the condoms and to the implied colors of various ethnic and racial groups featured in the clothing ads. The great playwright and poet Frederico Garcia Lorca wrote that "the eye is the processor of the senses" (Colombo, 1993, 74), a statement that sums up Toscani's aesthetic strategy. The eye is strategically drawn from left to right, the direction the Western eye is trained to travel when we read text. The condoms point to the right and the logo on the far right is the last thing the viewer observes. Even if we remember nothing about the picture, the logo will remain like a tattoo on our consciousness. The image of the bobbing condoms may be incomprehensible, but the familiar name will be retained and Benetton's commercial goal will have been met.

The condoms swim in a forward direction according to the common practices of looking. They appear to chase the open circles in a predatory act, and yet these latex receptacles hang suspended in midair, conspicuously lifeless and inert in their status as empty shells. Here again, Toscani challenges his viewer with mixed messages, or perhaps no message at all. The company has been categorical in its refusal to comment on any of the images it has produced. Interpretation and contextualization is left entirely up to the viewer in a distinctively postmodern refusal of narrative contingency. Critic Henry Giroux (1993) points out that postmodernism's (perhaps naive or even utopian) politics of questioning subjectivity and constructing identity as a social act has been easily co-opted by commerce: "If postmodern theory has used concepts such as the decentered subject or plural identities to analyze the emergence of broader cultural and social changes, mass market advertisers have seized upon the cultural logic of postmodernism to rearticulate politics and difference into the stylized world of aesthetics and consumption" (5–6).

Toscani's condom antics are no different. Though the condom is the sole available signifier in this ad, the referent is missing, absent from the message. That is, unless Benetton is surreptitiously selling condoms, or perhaps merely selling the "idea" of the condom. In the early nineties, condoms became a code word for the global politics of disease: AIDS. Benetton's condom image is not an ad for condoms *per se*, but it nevertheless capitalizes on the political correctness of promoting safe sex, all the while keeping the message ambiguous so as not to be seen as preaching a conservative attitude toward the use of the body. The various sizes, shapes, and colors of the condom continue Benetton's theme of difference and multivocality. And the muted, wallpaper-like banality of the image mocks the seriousness of the traditional campaigns around condom usage. In the end, the message retains its postmodern "playfulness."

Seduction: Coloring the Condom and Veiling the Body

In addition to Benetton's condom ad, the popular prophylactic is featured as the centerfold of its trendy youth magazine, *COLORS*. Here again, there are no bodies in sight but merely a collage of multicolored latex sheaths in all sorts of trendy colors and quirky forms. Each unique condom in the feature article entitled "Ready to Wear" is showcased in a larger-than-life photograph measuring a staggering foot and a half in height. The subtitle cautiously hints at the new importance of covering the male member but does not mention the disease in question by name: "Talking a man into wearing a condom is easy if you choose the right one. The right man. And the right condom" (1992, 3, 32).

Jean Baudrillard's concept of *seduction* will serve as a backdrop for an analysis of the social role of the condom and how it is featured in Benetton's images. In a post-Foucauldian sexual economy, where sexuality arises from a process of production, seduction is the ultimate denial of the "natural." In fact, it is the sign *par excellence* of artifice. Seduction is nothing but a veil, hiding the absent Lacanian Real or the Phallus, or even the Kantian "Ding-an-sich." It plays upon reversibility, irony, hyperreality, and above all, femininity: "The feminine seduces," Baudrillard (1990a) tells us, "because it is never where it thinks it is, or where it thinks itself" (6). Consequently, "the strength of the feminine is that of seduction" (7), for the feminine may be the object of the male gaze but it is also the controller of the gaze, manipulating it like a *trompe l'oeil*. Seduction is an unpredictable game, where surface is all that exists, a surface that masks and negates the possibility of authenticity and truth. Seduction is a simulation and a reversal of the real, always already an otherness of being, a powerful trope embodied in the neither/nor image of the transvestite. Ultimately, however, seduction is about the perverse desire to fascinate, tantalize, and dominate with the power of representation, fake or real.

From *se-ducere*, to take aside or divert from one's path, seduction is about desire, not pleasure. Pleasure is denied in the perpetual hallway of mirrors that leads the subject astray and keeps secrets hidden. Benetton's condom images function in much the same way to parade desire and thwart pleasure. They are all veil with nothing to show for it—the Phallus is an absent referent and its power has disappeared along with it. All that exists is a hollow shell, riddle, or toy, devoid of meaning, political or otherwise. Unlike Benetton's traditional advertisements, which showcase bodies and not clothing, the condoms featured here show nothing but the garment and banish the corporeal. This is a ready-to-wear garment without the model. The condom, like seduction, is a *trompe l'oeil*, making promises it cannot keep—promises of erotic or romantic encounters without the real-world referent of the material body and its mortality: "the *trompe-l'oeil*—falser than false—the secret of appearances....Simulacra without perspective, the figures in the *trompe-l'oeil* appear suddenly, with lustrous exactitude, as though denuded of the aura of meaning and bathed in ether" (60–61).

The funky, postmodern construction of sexuality in Benetton's cool, colorful condom spread is an apt analogy for Baudrillard's genealogy of the sign, which he outlines in four stages. The first is use-value, the natural stage, followed by the mercantile stage or exchange value, after which comes the structural stage, characterized by the code as sign-value. The fourth and final stage is what Baudrillard (1990b) calls the "fractal stage," the viral stage of negative-value and the end of reference (13). We can trace elements of all of these through Benetton's representation of condoms: Use-value is the element of protection, implied but not stated. Exchange-value is the condom as commodity to be bought and sold as a novelty item. Code- or sign-value is apparent in the elusive promise of erotic pleasure. More interesting, however, is Baudrillard's last phase, the fractal stage, whereby the signified is entirely removed from the condom as signifier, left as a limp veil, devoid of meaning-producing reference.

Each of the six full-page newspaper format images is accompanied by a caption telling a teasing story of the man who will potentially sport the rubber garment. The condom with the spiked, punk-hair pompom head has this text in the margin:

> For Helio, who you meet at the Earth summit in Rio. He is the one who won't use disposable coffee cups and instead carries his "Think Globally. Act Locally" ceramic mug. All those sad, beautiful stories he tells you about the rain forest. Tell him that this is made from pure Amazonian latex. Tell him that it's refillable. (*COLORS* 1992, 3, 33)

This terse caption is full of cliché and cynicism, where safe sex is paid the same lip service as token environmentalism, just one part of a hip, global lifestyle. Wearing a condom is likened to Helio's dogmatic opinions on recycling, albeit with a sarcastic edge: "It's refillable." We are invited to question whether we—or Helio, for that matter—can really save the Earth by printing catchy slogans on our personal accessories. In a rhetorical parallel, we are made to question the effectiveness of the condom against the global disaster of HIV/AIDS. Helio is painted as a hopeless romantic, nostalgic for simpler times, when values were real and old-growth forest was intact. His environmentalism is mocked by the speaker when he emphasizes the depletion of nonrenewable resources in the production of condoms. Will Helio refuse for this reason?

Another condom, the black licorice one with crocodile bumps, is "For Bjørn, who you meet on the beach in Jamaica. His skin is the color of strawberry soda pop. His blond hair is in dreadlocks. And he wants you to call him

Jah Warrior" (34) Like Helio's travel mug, Bjørn's dreadlocks symbolize his global lifestyle, but in the place of environmental consciousness is a concern with racial politics or perhaps merely a desire to appropriate racial otherness. Wearing a black condom vicariously inherits all the associations of colonial power mixed with sexual exoticism. Condoms here have reached Baudrillard's fractal stage of signification—they have no use-value and only *seduction* value in the sense of surface, *trompe-l'oeil*, and lifestyle accessory, where identity politics become just another a commodity.

One fundamental difference between the condoms featured in this *COLORS* article and those of Toscani's contentious Benetton ad is that these do not float in mute limbo but are accompanied by text in both English and Japanese, arguably two important languages of global culture.[5] The dialogue in the margins of the oversized condom spread brings these inert beings to life, anthropomorphizing them like puppets or low-maintenance pets. The sterility and clinical nature of the condom is removed as it becomes a humorous and benevolent presence, softening the jetlag of a fast-paced global existence. And yet we are not allowed to forget commodity culture—on the contrary, the feature article is tailored to remind us of a quality shopping experience and resembles an upscale catalogue to help us choose the perfect gift for that special someone. One such condom is topped with a grotesque gargoyle complete with beady eyes, horns, pointy ears and nose, and a protruding tongue. This one is for that someone you love to hate, a practical joke where the viewer is invited to partake in the pleasure of creating a victim. In this instance of dramatic irony, the author and the viewer are aware of the different levels of signification, but the butt of the joke is ignorant: "For Heinie, who you ditch near the Brandenburg Gate. Good riddance. You're better off without him" (36).[6] If Benetton celebrates racial otherness, here is an example where Heinie is demonized as a German and a member of the über-white race, guilty via his association with Nazi history. The messages and prejudices surrounding race, culture, and sexuality in Benetton's condom spread are layered and complex. Like a postmodern labyrinth, it is an impossible task to unravel and decipher them all. And that is exactly the point—they are meant to provoke and titillate, not to provide easy answers to global questions.

Full of associations to global lifestyle trends but emptied of either human flesh or use-value, these condom images beg the question: Whatever happened to the Lacanian Phallus as ultimate signifier to which all other signifiers refer in the process of meaning production? Whatever happened to the Phallus as a symbol of virile masculinity, noticeably absent from these pages? Instead, seduction, the feminine principle of uncertainty, uses the power of the veil to reverse and implode desire back upon itself—it becomes a self-seduction, a simulation of desire. "The male is no longer interesting," argues Baudrillard (1990a), "because too determined, too marked—the phallus as canonical signifier—and thus too fragile" (27). The ultimate irony here is that Benetton's image of the condom negates the masculine. Though associated with the penis, an ostensibly male organ, the condom featured here as a lifeless garment has been emasculated by the feminine principle of the veil.

Desire is a one-dimensional force and the fulfillment of desire is death. But seduction is reversible—every seduction is always already a self-seduction—and thus infinitely more powerful in its immortality. There is an element of narcissism present in the self-reflexive quality of the fractal stage, as witnessed in the empty condom, sheer veil, devoid of referent. Or as Baudrillard (1990a) puts it: "It is when signs are seduced that they become seductive" (74). Benetton's condoms arguably seduce themselves, demonstrating the reversibility of desire: seduction. Seen in these terms, the condom image is an analogy for Benetton's postmodern advertising strategies—the absent penis is like the absent product. The clothing items are missing from most of its ads just as the penis is the missing but connoted element behind the condom. The hidden message behind all of these images seems to be that the veil is all-powerful, all-signifying, and that in the end bodies do not matter.

Racial Harmony: Exoticism and the Cultural Other
Before coming back to this question, let us further examine the relationship between Benetton's representation of condoms and its carefully constructed statements about racial harmony. In its brochures and catalogues, Benetton presents us with young people of all different races and ethnicities, echoing the brightly colored garments featured. But the bodies themselves are highly uniform, anatomically correct in the age of semi-anorexic models. Thus the sameness of the bodies negates all the difference, albeit exoticized, celebrated through a multiplicity of races. Such images, claims Ian Roderick (1992), "promise a moment of contact with the cultural Other that is always harmonious. In order for the peoples to be united, there must be a corresponding moment of universalization or homogenization" (21). These bodies are what Douglas Coupland calls "global teens" in *Generation X*—regardless of their culture or country of origin, they have been raised in a world where global markets formulate their consumer habits.[7] Benetton's cloning mechanism produces difference and sameness simultaneously: different races, same

clothes, different faces, same bodies. Dark-skinned people appearing in advertising is a historical practice dating back to colonial times: "The production, consumption and commercialization of products were essential components of British imperialism," writes Jeffrey Auerbach (2002, 2). Auerbach demonstrates that five tropes—exoticization, racialization, sexualization, commodification, and civilization—developed as a form of propaganda to sell empire itself (3). Benetton seeks to appropriate this practice and disarm it through irony; however, it can well be argued that the company merely perpetuates already ingrained racial stereotypes.

The images of condoms fit into this same profile. The condoms are of all different sizes, shapes, and colors, thus mimicking Benetton's stated pursuit of racial harmony and the celebration of difference. They negate that very inclusiveness by masking the absent referent behind the pictures: AIDS and the specific suffering of peoples of color.[8] Race is a significant factor in the global pandemic of AIDS. Of the 40 million people worldwide infected with HIV, more than 62 percent of these cases are in Africa.[9] In Botswana, one of the worst affected areas, a shocking 37.3 percent of the adult population is currently infected with HIV. Even in the United States, where almost half a million people are currently infected, 66 percent of the cases are among people of color.[10] The situation has changed drastically since the early nineties when Benetton was producing its controversial ads and the current extent of the devastation in Sub-Saharan Africa could not have been predicted. Even given this fact, the insensitivity on the part of Benetton to the staggering problem that AIDS presents cannot be ignored.

Neither Benetton's condom ad nor the *COLORS* feature article mentions that condoms protect against sexually transmitted diseases including AIDS, and the images are all targeted at the company's main consumer base of moneyed, middle-class, European, predominantly white audiences, who do not see themselves as part of an at-risk population. The very people who most need the condoms—sex workers, intravenous drug users, people in poverty-stricken African countries—are economically excluded from participating in the dialogue between the image of the condom and the real condom (which is and is not a product). Benetton's flippant use of the condom image not only ignores disadvantaged, at-risk groups, but makes a mockery of them with its playful, postmodern aesthetic. Irony is a dominant trope of postmodernism, one that was quickly co-opted by clever advertisers keen to cash in on the power of tongue-in-cheek communication tactics. The condom ad that is not an ad for condoms capitalizes on this rhetorical mode, and yet, as Linda Hutcheon (1995) points out in *Irony's Edge*, irony always has a victim. Hutcheon tells us that the knife edge of irony is wielded against those who do not have the necessary information to attribute irony where it is intended. These victims, for whom irony is misunderstood or does not happen at all, are excluded and often embarrassed: "Many communication models of irony are based on the *necessity* of there being an excluded audience that does not understand the ironist's intention" (43). Whether intentional or not, the victims of Benetton's condom ads are those people who most need the condom and who are the least likely to benefit from the apparent altruism of these images.

For Benetton's target audience of white Europeans, the condom is just another consumer item, somewhat trendier than it used to be, precisely because it had become politically correct. Beginning in the mid-eighties with the onset of the first AIDS crisis, grassroots movements and community groups successfully lobbied governments to launch safe-sex education programs in schools and public health institutions, but also in bars and at public events. All of a sudden, it was not taboo to talk about condoms, and they began to appear on billboards and in promotional materials everywhere. They became party favors and door prizes and in some cases even replaced the after-dinner mint (Parisot, 1985, 112). Condoms had come out of the closet and were no longer the object of embarrassed laughter or restricted to a clinical environment.

Marketing Strategies: Protection vs. Pleasure
Even so, condom advertisement was not universally accepted, and it never has been. Vulcanized rubber condoms were first advertised in *The New York Times* in 1861, when "Dr. Power's French Preventatives" were marketed as contraceptive devices. However, this liberal period was short-lived, as the Comstock Law was passed in 1873 prohibiting the public display and promotion of all prophylactics.[11] Even today, advertisements are not commonly seen in magazines or other print media—while scantily clad women are welcome on the pages of most publications, the sight of a latex condom can still provoke negative reactions from conservative viewers. Even in youth, alternative, and scene magazines, editors are conscious of public sensibilities and do not want to offend or embarrass.[12] Ironically, menstruation does not fall into this category—ads for feminine hygiene products are commonplace on television and in print.

While North American condom producers have always stressed the health benefits of condoms in terms of prevention of pregnancy and sexually transmitted diseases, in the eighties a Japanese company named Kimono began making inroads into Western markets with a new product and a different message. This condom, made from polyurethane instead of latex, is thinner and well lubricated and the advertisements stressed pleasure and erotic potential with protection as an added bonus. With condoms as the major form of contraception in Japan (where hormonal drugs like the Pill are considered harmful to a woman's health), product design, packaging, and advertising is quite different. Accessories and gimmicks play a large role—you can buy condoms disguised as cigarette packs or cosmetic containers. Some packages play music when opened, others experiment with texture, shape, color, flavor, and scent, and some even come with handy disposal bags and wet wipes for easy clean-up (Parisot, 1985, 53–55).

Following their Japanese counterparts, American manufacturers saw the increased awareness of the health benefits of condom use as a commercial opportunity, and condom stores started sprouting up in major urban centers. The dramatic decline in condom use that began in the 1960s with the introduction of the Pill was quickly reversed in the 1980s by successful marketing on the part of both manufacturers and health organizations. Within a few years condoms came in every imaginable flavor and form—the lowly "safe" had achieved the status of sensual object or even sex toy. Despite this image makeover, the majority of condoms sold today are still dull "skin-toned" latex sheaths packaged in banal rectangular boxes.[13]

Studies show that changes to the actual condom in terms of width, thickness, and material seem to have little effect on the consumer. In other words, if someone does not like condoms, it will make no difference whether the condom is long and narrow, short and wide, thick or thin. Marketing, it would appear, is the only way to combat ignorance and indifference. While promotion of healthy choices is important and effective, the public will be even more enticed to wear condoms if they are told that condoms are sexy and increase erotic pleasure (Spruyt & Finger, 1998, 21). This is perhaps one of the good outcomes of Benetton's condom ads—they foster the view of condoms as sexy consumer objects rather than sterile medical apparatus. Here, postmodern playfulness no longer represents an offensive insensitivity to disadvantaged groups but becomes a successful strategy to influence public opinion. The problem remains, however, that at-risk groups are still unlikely to view these ads, placed in trendy fashion magazines and other elite publications.

Postscript: The Politics of Aesthetics

Benetton continued its wry humor and ironic messages with its cheeky proposal for a vast monument in the shape of a condom to be erected in St. Peter's Square in Vatican City. Featured in the fifth issue of *COLORS*, the article bordered on the ridiculous and was particularly offensive to Catholics. Though Benetton claims to treat all cultures, ethnicities, races, and faiths equally, the Italian company evidently feels at liberty to critique the dominant power structures in its own culture. *COLORS* editor Tibor Kalman complained that the Pope's message of abstinence is at best outdated and unrealistic, and at worst, dangerous. When asked if he was worried about offending the billion Catholics around the world, many of whom are Benetton customers, Kalman flatly denied any concern (Williams, 1994, 50). Clearly, Kalman, like Toscani, trusts his customers' judgment and their capacity to see the message beyond the ridicule.

What is interesting about Toscani's promotional endeavors is that he has succeeded in blurring the distinction among economics, aesthetics, and politics. Ads are essentially about achieving market success, but they spill over into the world of art—Toscani's images were exhibited at the Contemporary Art Museum in Pully-Lausanne and later at the Biennale of Venice in 1993. The creator of Benetton's hugely successful ad campaign no longer trades in the world of commerce alone but is viewed as an artist, whose creations merit serious analysis. It is telling that Toscani's photographs were exhibited without Benetton's trademark green logo. The boundaries between art and commerce may be blurred, but they have not been eradicated.[14]

Seen as pure aesthetic creations, however, Toscani's condom creations are dangerously displaced from a grave reality. In a world where it seems as though representation is all that matters, the condom is no longer real but a simulation, to use Baudrillard's terminology. In his self-consciously postmodern style, Toscani's condoms are already doubles of themselves. Their use-value has disappeared along with the referent, and the image is all that counts. The condom refers not to the receptacle worn on the erect male member, but to another colorful sheath and another and another.

Oliviero Toscani is aware of the tremendous importance of establishing value as experienced through the eye, a view that reflects W. J. T. Mitchell's (2002) theory that "the relationship between images and value is among the central issues of contemporary criticism" (1). Iconology and mediology speak to the "pictorial turn" as the postmodern follow-up of Richard Rorty's "linguistic turn" (Mitchell, 2002, 2). Images are distinct from pictures, where pictures are the raw materials and images equal the sum total of the interaction of the picture with social discourse, cultural context, and the viewer's horizon of expectations. While pictures are concrete objects, images are ethereal conglomerates of mental and psychological processes. This means that no matter what the criteria for analysis, we cannot disentangle the "artistic value" of Benetton's ads from their commercial and political value.

My point here is that the ads cannot be viewed exclusively as an economic medium or artistic expression but are also highly politicized. Toscani may have aspirations to become recognized as a master photographer and publicity genius, but Benetton's stated position is that its primary concern is political and social. Having made grand claims to altruistic motives, the company must recognize the responsibility of its influence on erotic communities and sexual economies. In their stalwart refusal to interpret or preach, Benetton's condom ads straddle the edges of postmodern representational practices. On the one hand, they manufacture and appropriate political correctness to their benefit, and on the other hand they attempt to shock the public out of complacency around HIV and AIDS. The marriage of corporate and philanthropic goals is a complicated one, and Benetton has been accused, rightly or not, of capitalizing on the suffering of others. And yet in placing condoms and other taboo subjects on billboards and other public venues, Benetton is perhaps a leader in a new sexual revolution, one that moves beyond the nostalgia and romance of "free sex," beyond the syntax of morality, and toward the sexiness of safe sex. Like the cagey seduction of the veil, the condom in these ads refers infinitely and only to its own devices, be they medical, technological, or erotic.

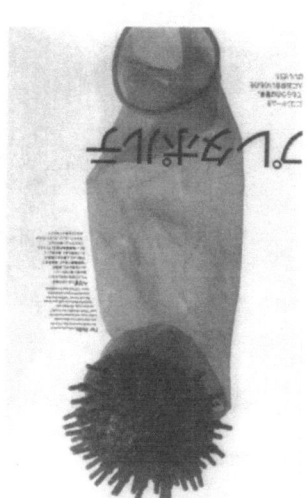

For Helio, Benetton clothing ad.

222 • The Colors of the Condom •

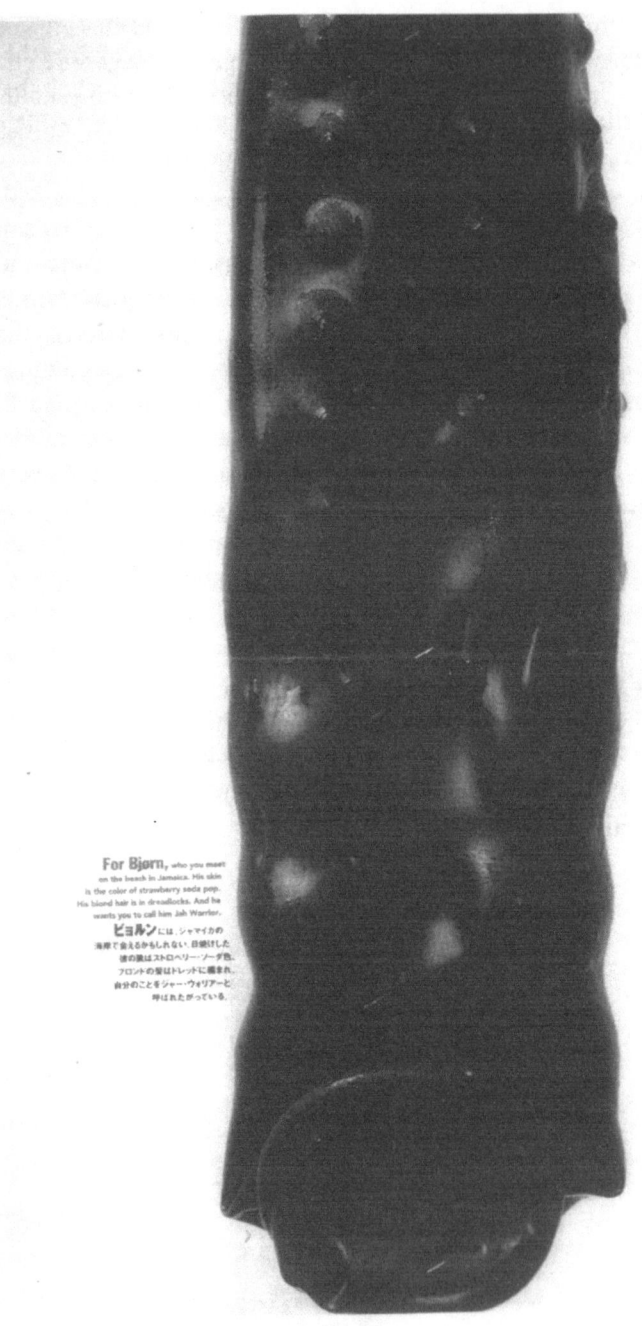

For Bjorn, Benetton clothing ad.

The Colors of the Condom

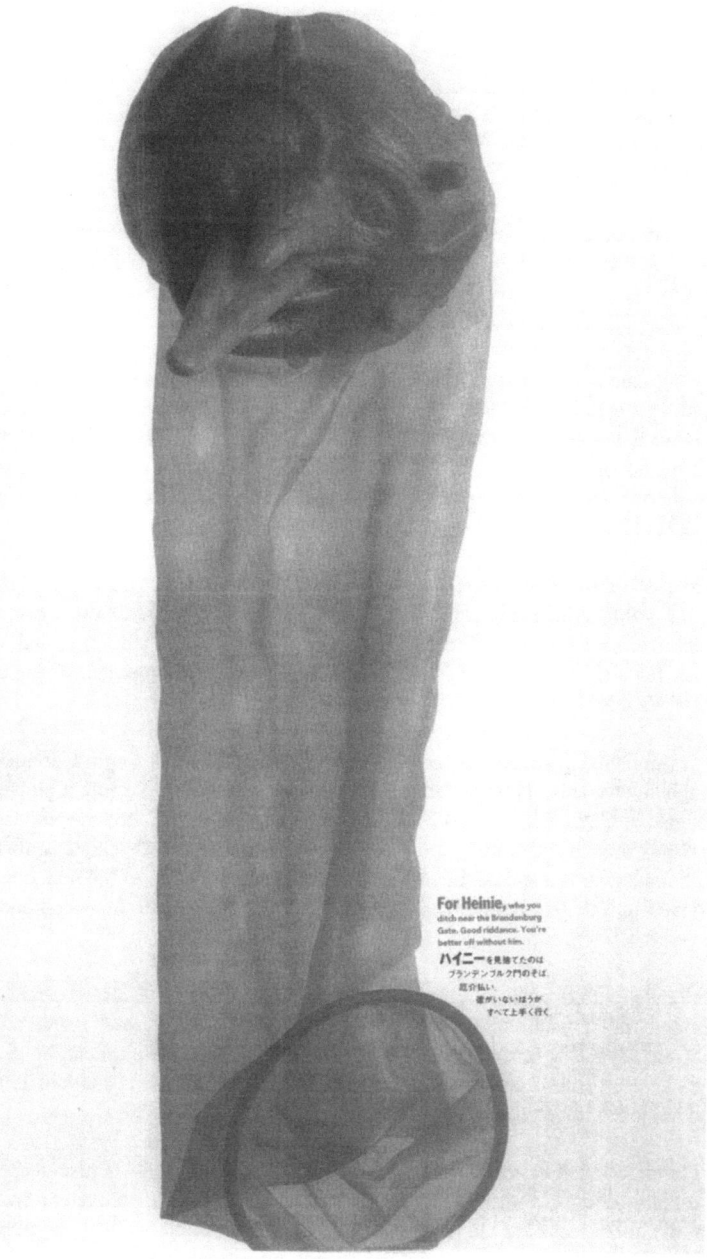

For Heine, Benetton clothing ad.

Notes

[1] For Jacques Lacan, the "Phallus" is the focus of desire and has nothing to do with the male organ of the penis. The Phallus is a social construct that organizes power as the object of desire. It is also the ultimate signifier against which all other signifiers take on meaning (see Gallop, 1982, 127–156).

[2] In Lacan's terminology, the "real" serves a function of constancy and cannot be expressed in language. It is elusive and always just beyond reach of comprehension. The real is juxtaposed to the "imaginary," which corresponds to language in an ideal state, and the "symbolic," which is the use of language that enables subjectivity (Jirgens, 1993, 397).

[3] Douglas Coupland's *Generation X* features a chapter entitled "I am not a target market," which pinpoints a certain trend among populations to avoid identifying with a group of any kind. This is what I would call a postmodern addiction to authenticity—the emphasis on difference as a means of constructing a unique subjectivity. The irony is that this very group—those who choose not to belong to a target market—is Benetton's target market (see Coupland, 1991, 17–22).

[4] Founded in 1991 with the rather self-centered title *COLORS: A Magazine about the Rest of the World*, the publication made a public mission statement: "All over the world Benetton stands for colorful sportswear, multiculturalism, world peace, racial harmony, and a progressive approach toward serious social issues" (*COLORS* Spring/Summer, 5). These are rather lofty goals for what is ostensibly a catalogue with a few articles.

[5] *COLORS* is published in several different bilingual editions: French/English, Italian/English, Japanese/English, etc. This is just one more means of inviting the reader into a global community. The magazine *COLORS* still exists and has come out with more controversial issues such as one on prisons around the world. However, the circulation and readership is now relatively small and the magazine is a special interest publication on the fringes of the mainstream. Benetton has moved into the background as a retailer and as an acteur in the social and political arena.

[6] Each condom is paired with a fictional character who is ridiculed for a certain character trait—environmentalist, wannabe Rastafarian, German—but mostly these figures are mocked for their naïveté regarding serious social and political issues. The implication is that only someone as naive as Helio, Bjørn, or Heinie would think that such a condom is really for wearing and not just a novelty item.

[7] "Global Teens" is another term coined by Douglas Coupland, who is also responsible in large part for the term "Generation X," which has now become a permanent word in our global lexicon. Global teens are the first generation of well-traveled, well-to-do young people, for whom citizenship is immaterial. They are shaped by international trends, most of which

originate in Europe and North America. They are first and foremost consumers, the type Benetton most wants to target. In his later book, *Shampoo Planet,* Coupland (1992) refines and specifies the term further, coining the phrase "Benetton Youth."

[8] It is impossible to discuss Benetton's representation of condoms without reference to its representation of AIDS in the same ad campaign. These images were perhaps the most disagreeable to the public of all Benetton's ads. One such ad featured AIDS patient David Kirby on his deathbed surrounded by his family. Another disturbing image was a picture of the inside of a man's forearm tattooed with the letters "HIV," making obvious reference to the scars of intravenous drug-users. Benetton was accused of profiting from the suffering of others by making a public spectacle of their pain, and of creating stereotypes around the disease of AIDS and drug abuse.

[9] See *www.avert.org/aafrica.htm*. AVERT is a leading UK-based AIDS Education and Medical Research charity, which carries out a wide range of education and medical research work. Their mandate involves the prevention of HIV infection, improving the quality of life for those infected, and working toward a cure for AIDS. Statistics around AIDS change at such a rapid pace that the Internet is often the most reliable source. Numbers and facts are sometimes outdated by the time they are published in print.

[10] Benetton's representation of AIDS through images of condoms documents early misperceptions in terms of at-risk groups. It was assumed that men would make up the majority of AIDS victims because it appeared that the disease was linked to the gay community, intravenous drug users, and prison inmates. This picture has reversed itself such that married women are perhaps even more at risk than men. Women are more susceptible to infection, and men are less likely to wear a condom in a conjugal relationship. Women are nowhere to be seen in representations of AIDS in the early nineties and are still seldom pictured as typical victims.

[11] See *www.avert.org/condoms.htm*. Germany passed a similar law in 1922, making condom ads illegal, and during the Second World War, rubber was in such short supply in Britain that there were calls to stop the production and sale of condoms "in the interest of national welfare" (Parisot, 1985, 39). In 1959 condom vending machines were prohibited in Germany, and so they were banished to men's lavatories (not considered public) until 1970, when the law was overturned.

[12] The only place where condoms are regularly advertised in my community is on the local rock radio station, perhaps because this is a purely acoustic medium and therefore neatly skirts the whole issue of visual representation. In North America, even condom packaging itself does not commonly display the contents.

[13] In recent years, technical improvements, increased reliability, and innovations in marketing and design have contributed to the new image, and yet there are still many obstacles to be overcome in ensuring widespread, global use of the condom: perceived unreliability as protection against pregnancy and disease; many people do not believe they are at risk; couples are

too embarrassed or worry about their partner's reaction at the suggestion of using condoms; lack of skill; lack of communication between sex workers and their clients; limited availability in some areas of the world; cultural and political norms that reinforce negative perceptions of the condom. These are all serious concerns for medical professionals and health organizations; however, recent studies suggest that the single most important obstacle to overcome is that consumers do not like them (Lewis, 1998, 2). Separate research in Jamaica and China indicates that both men and women name among their chief reasons for not using condoms that they reduce sensation and that they inhibit spontaneity. There is also a common misconception that they break easily or that sperm can pass through the membrane (Spruyt & Finger, 1998, 13). Among married women of reproductive age, only 5 percent use condoms on a regular basis and only 3 percent in less developed regions (Spruyt & Finger, 1998, 12). However, it has equally been shown that consistent health promotion has a significant effect on use. In Haiti, for example, such a marketing campaign increased condom sales twofold in a four-year period. And in Nepal, sales more than doubled within three years (Spruyt & Finger, 1998, 15).

[14] Toscani's carefully polished photographs were displayed with no documentation showing the evolutionary process from raw photograph to final image—we learn nothing of the context or subjects.

Bibliography

Auerbach, J. (2002). Art, advertising, and the legacy of empire. *Journal of Popular Culture, 35*(4): 1–24.

Baudrillard, J. (1990a). *Seduction.* (Trans. by B. Singer) Montreal: New World Perspectives.

———. (1990b). *La Transparence du mal: Essai sur les phénomènes extrêmes.* Paris: Galillée.

Colombo, F. (1993). Advertising, naked, and fully clothed + Benetton. *Aperture,* 132: 74–75.

COLORS: A magazine about the rest of the world. (1992). Number 3, 33–37.

Coupland, D. (1991). *Generation X: Tales for an accelerated culture.* New York: St. Martin's Press.

———. (1992). *Shampoo planet.* New York: Simon and Schuster.

Finkelstein, J. (1991). *The fashioned self.* Cambridge: Polity Press.

Gallop, J. (1982). *The daughter's seduction: Feminism and psychoanalysis.* Ithaca, NY: Cornell University Press.

Giroux, H. (1993). Consuming social change: The united colors of Benetton. *Cultural Critique,* 25: 5–32.

Hutcheon, L. (1995). *Irony's edge.* New York: Routledge.

Jirgens, K. (1993). Lacan. In I. R. Makaryk (Ed.), *Encyclopedia of contemporary literary theory* (pp. 396–398). Toronto: University of Toronto Press.

Langman, L. (1992). Neon cages: Shopping for subjectivity. In R. Shields (Ed.), *Lifestyle shopping: The subject of consumption.* London: Routledge.

Lewis, J. (1998). Why a monograph on latex condoms? In E. T. McNeill et al. (Eds.), *The latex condom: Recent advances, future directions* (pp. 2–4). NP: Family Health International.

Mitchell, W. J. T. (2002). The surplus value of images. *Mosaic,* 35(3): 1–23.

O'Leary, N. (1992). Benetton's true colors. *Adweek,* 24 August: 27–31.

Parisot, J. (1985). *Johnny come lately: A short history of the condom.* London: Journeyman.

Roderick, I. (1992). What is it that unites the colors of Benetton? *Fuse,* 15: 21–23.

Sischy, I. (1992). Advertising taboos: Talking to Luciano Benetton and Oliviero Toscani. *Interview,* April: 68–71.

Spruyt, A., & Finger, W. (1998). Acceptability of condoms: Use behaviors and product attributes. In E. T. McNeill et al. (Eds.), *The latex condom:*

Recent advances, future directions (pp. 12–21). NP: Family Health International.

Squiers, I. (1992). Violence at Benetton and the socially conscious and outrageous ad campaigns. *Artforum, 30*(9): 18–19.

Williams, H. A. (1994). Voice of colors: Tibor Kalman. *Graphis, 50*(291): 50–51.

Willis, S. (1983). Disney World: Public use/private state. *The South Atlantic Quarterly, 92*(1): 119–138.

• CHAPTER SEVENTEEN •

Condom Flowers

Angelika Foerst

In 1974, in response to Thailand's high volume of sex trade (the prostitution of women and young boys), and in an effort to curb the country's annual growth rate, the Population and Community Development Association (PDA), founded by Senator Mechai Viravaidya, was created. Otherwise known as "Mr. Condom," Senator Viravaidya and the PDA organized communities and rural development projects ranging in purposes from environmental protection to HIV/AIDS education.

Viravaidya's contention was that by using the condom to symbolize his family planning campaign, he would thus elicit strong reactions, and once these feelings were acknowledged and then voiced, Thais would be prepared to listen to his message on safe-sex education. It was likewise Mechai Viravaidya's position that condoms ought to be as easily accessible to the public as vegetables in a grocery store. This condom crusader, fighting against HIV and poverty, has worked for forty years toward the economic and social development of Thailand; thereby lending his name (Mechai-Mechais) to these pocket (-sized) protectors.

In order to remove the stigma attached to speaking about condom usage, Viravaidya and the PDA had to transform the mentality of Thais, getting them to breathe, sleep, and eat condoms. For this reason, they established Cabbages and Condoms Bangkok, an eatery that offers its patrons a condom in lieu of the traditional mint following their *bon repas*, giving new meaning to the phrase *bon appetit*. Tabletops adorned with glass-encased rubbers, bouquets made from contraceptives, and condom cartooned carpets represent its daily decor.

The population of Thailand is 60,609,000. All of the efforts taken to inform the public have resulted in a "dramatic drop in the Thai birth rate from 3.2% to 1.1%" (Trinity Today, 2002–2003: 2). In order to promote safe sex, the sex workers of Thailand hand-make the condom flowers found in these restaurants. These handmade crafts not only serve to provide an alternative income, but they also enable these "artists" to care for their families.

Despite celebrating World AIDS Day for twenty years, 14,000 new HIV infections occur on a daily basis. In recognition of this devastating statistic, the Burnet Institute of Australia purchases these condom bouquets in order to help raise awareness and funds that will support its work in the International Health area. The profits for the Thai condom flowers sold in Australia are then channeled into HIV prevention and education programs run by the institute, all in the effort to care for the 13 million vulnerable young children orphaned as a result of their parents having contracted AIDS. The quest is to conquer the taboo associated with condoms, as well as to democratize their usage.

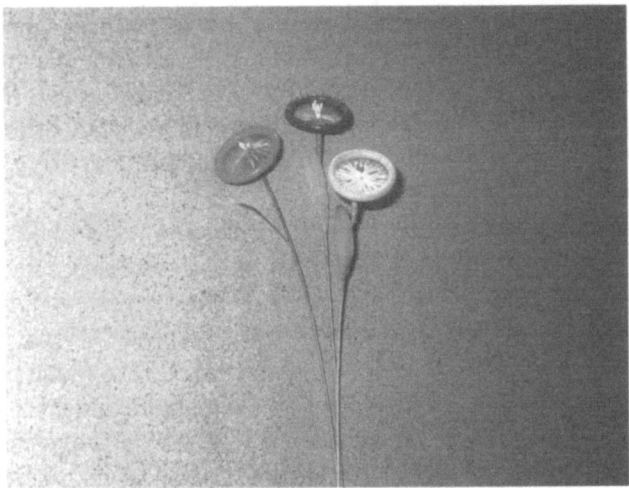

Condom Flowers sold by the Burnet Institute in Australia.

Bibliography

Internet site: *www.burnet.edu.au/about/media/10226.*

Internet site: *www.trinity.unimelb.edu.au/publications/trinitytoday/ summer02/mainevent25.shtml.*

Internet site: *www.unsociety .unsw.edu.au/UNtoday/cc.htm.*

Internet site: *www.gaia-s.net/SouthAsia2000/Notes/Thailand.html.*

Internet site: *www.inq7.net/opi/2003/oct/12/opi_rjdavid-1.htm.*

• CONTRIBUTORS •

Peter McLaren is professor of education at the Graduate School of Education and Information Studies, University of California at Los Angeles. His works cover subjects ranging from traditional schooling to media and popular culture and education as a revolutionary act. He is among the leading critical pedagogists in North America.

Karen Anijar is associate professor of curriculum and cultural studies at Arizona State University. She is the author of *Teaching Toward the 24th Century: Star Trek as Social Curriculum*.

Thuy DaoJensen is a doctoral candidate completing her dissertation in curriculum and cultural studies at Arizona State University. As a Spencer Foundation Dissertation Fellow, her dissertation will focus on abstinence-only sex educators and curriculum.

Jessamyn Neuhaus is assistant professor at Denison University and author of *Manly Meals and Mom's Home Cooking: Cookbooks and Gender in Modern America*.

Mary M. Dalton is assistant professor of communication at Wake Forest University, where she teaches film studies courses. Her research interest is critical media studies, documentaries, and screenwriting.

Chris Bell is a doctoral candidate in disability studies at University of Illinois at Chicago.

James H. Sanders is visiting associate professor in the College of Arts and Sciences' Department of Art Education at Ohio State University in Columbus. He is concurrently serving as coordinator of National Art Education Association's Caucus on Social Theory and Art Education.

Michael J. Nanna is a faculty associate in the College of Education at Arizona State University-East.

Mark Lipton is assistant professor in the School of English and Theatre Studies at the University of Guelph.

Devon C. Adams is a doctoral candidate completing his dissertation in curriculum studies at Arizona State University. His research interests include cultural studies, curriculum studies, gifted education, and advanced placement programs.

Charla Triplett holds an M.S. in bioengineering from Oregon State University and is currently pursuing her Ph.D in educational leadership and policy studies at Arizona State University.

Dacia Charlesworth (Ph.D., Southern Illinois University at Carbondale) is the director of the Office of Honors Programs and assistant professor of communications at Robert Morris University in Moon Township, PA. Charlesworth's research interests encompass rhetorical and performative intersections of gender/ethnicity/class, communication across the curriculum, and outcomes assessment.

Janis Faye Hutchinson is a medical anthropologist in the Department of Anthropology, University of Houston. Her research interests include condom use, HIV/AIDS, racism and health, and health issues among African Americans. Her publications focus on these topics and African-American identity as shown in her book *Cultural Portrayals of African Americans: Creating an Ethnic/Racial Identity*, 1997.

Vern L. Bulluogh is a SUNY dstinguished professor emeritus and founded the Center for Sex Research at California State University, Northridge. He is the author, co-author, or editor of more than fifty books, about half of which deal with sex and gender issues.

Ahmed Afzal is visiting assistant professor in the department of Sociology and Anthropology at Colgate University.

Jill Scott is assistant professor in the Department of German at Queen's University, Canada. She has published in the areas of cultural studies and German and comparative literature. She has recently published a book on the Electra myth in twentieth-century literature and culture, *Electra after Freud: Myth and Culture* (Cornell University Press, 2005).

Angelika Foerst is a doctoral candidate in curriculum and cultural studies at Arizona State University. Her research interests include queer theory, whiteness, youth and violence, and popular culture.

• INDEX •

•A•

ABCs of birth control, 173
Abstinence-based education, 1–15
Abstinence-only curriculum, 21–26
Abstinence, Africa, AIDS, 6
Action Fund, 105
Adlard, Carole, 11
Advocate, The, 33
African-American women, 131–154
AIDS, 1–8, 13, 21–23, 32, 42–44, 50, 51–55, 59, 65, 77, 80, 83, 101–103, 110, 117–126, 131, 142, 150–154, 163, 174–175, 178, 193, 197–198, 207, 209, 212, 217–218, 221, 229–230
Alexander, Jane, 62
Alfred C. Kinsey Institute, 77–79, 87
Allen, Claude, 11–12
Allen, Ted, 29
American Life League, 5
Andy Warhol Museum, 105
Ansell Limited, 79
Arts in education, 59–64
Ashcroft, John, 5–6, 16
Astruc, Johannes, 100–101
At-risk, 217, 219
Atwood, Margaret, 2

•B•

Baker v. State, 34
Bangkok World, 172–173
Barebacking, 102
Baudrillard, Jean, 207, 213–215, 220
Benetton clothing ads, 207–221
Benetton, Luciano, 211
Bernstein, E.L., 97
Bertini, Adriana, 163–168
Birth control pill, 90
Brazil, 163
Burnet Institute, 230
Bush, George, 4

•C•

Cabbages and Condoms, 169–175, 229–230
Casanova de Seingalt, Jacques, 100
Castration, 23–26
Cannery Row, 38
Censorship, 66
Centers for Disease Control (CDC), 22, 50, 56, 117–118
Choosing the Best curriculum, 13–14
Clinton administration, 4, 62
Cobb County, 7
COLORS magazine, 207–221
Community Based Family Planning Services, 172
Compton, Bishop Henry 99
Comstock law, 218
Condom flowers, 229–230
Condom King, The, 169–175

Condom roulette, 22
Condomania, 61, 88–91
Construction of condom use, 131–154
Coward, Rosalind, 111
Charles II, 99
Chicago Tribune, 56
Christian Right, 8, 22
Church of England, 99
Citizens for Excellence in Education, 10
Cold War, 26
Comedy Central, 37
Contemporary Art and Multicultural Education, 63
Coupland, Douglas, 216
Cultural studies, 61–68
  visual, 61–68
Culture Wars, 62, 66
Cyberspace, 109

•D•

Darwin, Charles, 88
Delderfield, Eric, 99
Democrats, 4
Designing Women, 55
Dewey, John, 62
Douglas, Kyan, 29, 33
Dr. Condon, 99
Durex, 77

•E•

Evita, 56
Education Defense Act, 62
Elementary and Secondary Education Act, 62

Engineers, 109–114

•F•

Fallopius, Gabrielle, 96–98
Family Research Council, 21–22
Female condom, 112–113
Female identity, 131–154
Female Health Foundation, 113
Feminism and Sexuality, 111
Fight Club, 113
Filicia, Thom, 29–32
Food and Drug Administration, 110
Foster, Mike, 3
French letters, 98
Freud, Sigmund, 24–26

•G•

GAPA , 163
Gardner, Howard, 61
Gay bashing, 33
Gender role theory, 153
Georgia, 7
Generation X, 90, 216
Giroux, Henry, 61, 212
Goals 2000, 62
Goodyear and Hancock, 90, 101
Goldwyn, Tony, 55
Government brochures, 117–127
Grease, 106
Grauman's Chinese Theater, 1

•H•

Hall, Stuart, 23

Hayes, Isaac, 44
Helms, Jesse, 62
Herrnstein, Richard, 68
Himes, N., 94, 97, 99–101
HIV, 6, 13, 22–23, 32, 41, 50, 54–55, 58–59, 65, 77, 90, 101–102, 110, 112, 117, 122–123, 125–126, 131–133, 135–136, 138, 142, 144, 147, 149–153
HIV testing, 150–153
Hirsh, Jodi, 107
Homosexuality, 33–34, 96, 102, 199
Homosociality, 195
Homophobia, 30, 33–34
House Committee on Un-American Activities, 62
Houston, 132–133
Hutcheon, Linda, 217–218

•I•

IMF, 192
Imperial Rome, 95–96
India, 84–86
Infidelity, 139, 143–144, 151
Inspiral condom, 111–112
In Living Color, 49
Irvine, Janice, 21

•J•

Jackson, Janet, 53, 55
Jeremiah Productions, 1–2

•K•

Kaiser Family Foundation, 11
KamaSutra condom, 192–193
Kelly-Mast, Colleen, 11
Killer Condom, 21–26
Kimmel, Michael, 34
Kimono, 218
Kressley, Carson, 29–30, 32

•L•

Lacanian symbol, 207
Lacanian phallus, 215
Langman, Lauren, 209
Latex, 22, 90–91, 93–94, 101–102, 110, 112–113, 163, 212, 214, 218–219
Lawrence v. Texas, 34
Lesbians, 31, 34
Lifeway Christian Resources, 8
Lopez, Jennifer, 38
Lorca, Frederico Garcia, 211
Louganis, Greg, 54

•M•

Marcuse, Herbert, 60
Marketing of condoms, 87, 109, 113, 218–219
Marxist analysis, 10
Masculinity, 19, 24–26
Mason, Anne, 230
Matrisciana, Caryl, 2
Matrisciana, Patrick, 2
Mazzarella, William, 192–193
McCarthy, Joseph, 5

Medical Institute for Sexual Health, 21
Metrosexual, 29
Michael, George, 54
Ministry of Health and Family Welfare, 183
Ministry of Population Welfare, 183–184, 188–191
Minos, 95–96
Miss Universe, 170
Monroe, Marilyn, 105–106
Morris, Marilyn, 11
MTV, 109
Multiple intelligences, 61
Murray, Charles, 78

•N•

NEA, 62, 66
NGO, Non-Government Organization, 173
No Child Left Behind, 68
No Second Chance, 1
Normal distribution, 78–81, 84–85

•O•

Orwell, George, 2
Oprah Winfrey show, 29
Outbreak, 1

•P•

Pakistan, 177–198
Pasiphaë, 95–96
Penis size, 77–91

Performance art, 59
Phallus, 207, 213, 215–216
Planned Parenthood, 105–107, 171–172
Population and Community Development Association, 174
Poseidon, 99–100
Post-fordist Puritanism, 5–6
Postmodern theory, 207, 212–221
Polyurethane, 91, 112, 218–220
Procris, 95–96, 102
"Proper Condom Use" episode, 37–47
Punjabi men, 178–180, 196–197

•Q•

Quality control, 163
Queer Eye for the Straight Guy, 29–34

•R•

Racial harmony, 208, 210, 216–217
Rap music, 50, 57, 132–133
Rational/scientific approach, 119, 123
Reality TV, 29–34
Re-Animator, The, 89
Red rocket game, 38–39, 47
Rich, B. Ruby, 62
Ricki Lake show, 53
Roderick, Ian, 216
Rodriguez, Jai, 29, 31
Rofes, Eric, 67
Romans, 96
Rorty, Richard, 220

· Index ·

Rosenfield, Allan, 171
Russian roulette, 13, 22

·S·

Safe sex, 3, 13, 21–23, 60, 106–107, 117, 124, 141
Salt-N-Pepa, 50, 55, 57
Same-sex sexual desire, 177, 179–180, 185, 193, 195–198
Sathi condom, 177–198
Sex,
    anal, 5, 119–121, 124
    education, 21–22, 37, 40–41, 43, 46–47
    oral, 5
    revolution, 90, 102, 221
Sex Respect curriculum, 8
Sexually transmitted diseases (STDs), 11, 32, 40, 45, 51, 90, 171
Sexually transmitted infections (STIs), 94, 103
Shaft, 44, 106
Shepherd, Linda, 109
Simonds, Robert, 10
Simpson, Mark, 29
Scopes monkey trial, 7
Social responsibility, 209–211
Some Like It On, 105–106
South Park, 37–47
Southeastern Surface Design Association Symposium, 64
SPAM e-mail, 89
Sputnik, 62
Standardization, 87
Statistical analysis, 77–87
Stiff Competition, 105–107
Steinbeck, John, 38

Sullivan, Kathleen, 8

·T·

Taylor, Frederick, 87
Taylor, Gary, 24–25
Tensile properties test, 111
Thailand, 169–175, 229–230
TLC, 49, 55
Toole, Mike, 230
Tonight Show, The, 29
Toscani, Oliviero, 210–212, 215, 220–221
True Love Waits, 8–10
    pledge, 9
Trojan
    condom, 15, 109
    horse, 15
Tueth, Michael, 38
Turner, Daniel, 98

·U·

Unruh, Leslee, 11
United National Population Award, 165
Unsafe sex, 62, 136, 141–145, 154
Urdu, 177, 181, 194–195

·V·

Vatican City, 219
Viravaidya, Mechai, 169–175, 229–230
Vulcanized rubber, 90, 218

•W•

Wakeman, Henry, 99
Wagner, David, 8
Walz, Martin, 23
Wisconsin Pharmacal, 102
Women's clothing, 163
World AIDS Day, 229
World Health Organization, 117

World War I, 90
World War II, 32, 90

•Z•

Z-distribution, 70
Zeus, 96